The TAO
of
Healing
Myasthenia Gravis

Self-Healing and Self-Help

STEPHEN LAU

Copyright © 2020 Stephen Lau
All rights reserved.
ISBN: 9781098994181

All the quotes from Lao Tzu are taken from the author's own book:
**The Complete TAO TE CHING
in Plain English**.

CONTENTS

	THE INTRODUCTION	7
ONE	THE KNOWLEDGE	9
TWO	THE WISDOM	21
THREE	THE TAO	41
FOUR	THE JOURNEY	49
	APPENDIX A:	191
	THE AUTHOR'S OWN HEALING JOURNEY	
	APPENDIX B:	201
	ABOUT THE AUTHOR	

THE INTRODUCTION

Millions and billions of people worldwide are suffering from autoimmune diseases, including *myasthenia gravis* which is only one of the many different autoimmune disorders that are causing anxiety, fear, pain, mental confusion, and even suicidal thoughts in some of those afflicted.

According to Western medicine, there is no known cure for autoimmune diseases due to the complexity of their causes. Understandably, patients afflicted with autoimmune diseases are seeking healing from many different healing modalities, such as the Traditional Chinese Medicine (TCM), the Ayurvedic medicine, and among many others. In addition, they are desperately looking for help from herbs, fruits, and all kinds of natural nutrient supplements, as well as from physical exercises and spiritual practices, to rejuvenate their failing health due to their weakened immune systems.

The TAO may play a pivotal role in the healing process of any autoimmune disease, including that of *myasthenia gravis*.

The TAO is the profound wisdom of **Lao Tzu**, the ancient sage from China more than 2,600 years ago, who was the author of the immortal ancient classic **Tao Te Ching** on human wisdom.

The word "TAO" (道) in Chinese originally meant "road." Later, it came to mean "way" and hence "the Way." The TAO is "the Way" of looking at the world with a certain attitude of the mind, which is totally different from that of the West, and that is why it is so intriguing and fascinating, as evidenced by the fact that *Tao Te Ching* (道 德 經), the book of the TAO by Lao Tzu, is one of the most translated books in the world.

The TAO may provide self-inspiration and self-intuition for those who have to confront all the changes and challenges when diagnosed with *myasthenia gravis* or any autoimmune disease.

Stephen Lau

ONE

THE KNOWLEDGE

The Trauma

If you or your loved ones have been diagnosed with *myasthenia gravis*, it must have been a devastating experience, especially if the neurologist has said that there is no known cure, except using medications to control and manage the many debilitating disease symptoms associated with *myasthenia gravis*.

A traumatic experience may have a prolonged effect on the human mind: having overwhelming negative emotions; feeling numb and unable to experience pleasure or even pain over a long period of time. The ultimate impact is that it may affect how you *think*, *feel*, *act*, and *react* in every aspect of your daily life and living.

To heal yourself of *myasthenia gravis* or any illness, you must be both *knowledgeable* and *wise*.

Knowledge and Wisdom

Knowledge comes from *how* your mind perceives and processes any information available. Wisdom, on the other hand, is how you *apply* the knowledge acquired to cope with any disease and disorder you may have, as well as your everyday life and living. The important implication: being knowledgeable may not necessarily make you wise or wiser.

The bottom line: you need *both* knowledge and wisdom to heal yourself of *myasthenia gravis*.

Given that both knowledge and wisdom come from the thinking mind, your brain is, therefore, the most important of all your body organs. With its billions of brain cells, your brain is not only most complicated but also major source of all your health issues and problems related to *myasthenia gravis*.

So, it is important to keep your brain healthy as much as possible in order to be capable of acquiring the knowledge and attaining the wisdom to heal your *myasthenia gravis*.

The Healthy Brain

This is *how* you may keep your brain healthy:

- Keep yourself hydrated because 80 percent of your brain is water. Drink at least 7-8 cups of water per day.

- Keep healthy gums, and floss your teeth regularly to prevent any gum disease.

- Enhance and improve blood flow to your brain with your 30-minute exercise at least several times a week.

- Eat a healthy diet: high-quality lean protein; low-glycemic and high-fiber carbohydrates; natural and not processed foods.

- Avoid inflammation and the formation of free radicals in your body.

- Avoid sugar and sugary drinks, including all sodas and diet sodas.

- Quit smoking, and limit your alcohol consumption to no more than 5 glasses per week.

- Manage your blood pressure, blood sugar and cholesterol levels.

- Maintain healthy levels of nutrients, e.g. vitamin D and omega-3s.

- Maintain healthy hormones of the thyroid and the testosterone.

- Promote good mental health, and avoid anxiety and depression.

- De-stress yourself with correct breathing and daily meditation.

- Get quality sleep of at least 7-8 hours a night without the help of medication.

- Develop meaning and purpose in your life.

In addition to having a healthy brain, you must learn how to *empower* your thinking mind to seek and acquire the knowledge to heal your *myasthenia gravis*.

The Questions and the Answers

Asking many relevant questions and seeking the answers from those questions asked is the way to *empower* your thinking mind.

There is an old proverb that says: "He who cannot ask cannot live." Life is all about asking questions and seeking answers from the questions asked—and *that* is empowering the human mind for knowledge and information.

After a devastating *myasthenia gravis* diagnosis, it is not uncommon for the patient to ask the question: "Why?" Asking this pivotal question can have either a negative or a positive impact on the patient. The question "Why *me*?" often leads to negative emotions, such as anger, anxiety, frustration, hopelessness, and even unfairness; while the question "*Why* do I have *myasthenia gravis*?" may result in the intent to do something positive about the causes of the disorder, leading to healing.

In the Bible, **Jesus** said: "Ask, and it shall be given you; seek, and ye shall find" (**Matthew** 7:7) In real life, we must always ask ourselves many thought-provoking questions at all times. Asking questions is self-introspection, which is a positive process of self-intuition and self-reflection, without which there is no self-awareness and hence no personal growth and development. Therefore, asking questions is self-empowering the thinking mind to get the knowledge, which is a tool necessary for any healing process.

Remember, the kind of questions you ask determines the kind of life you are going to live. Your questions often trigger a set of mental answers, which may lead to actions or inactions, based on the choices you are going to make from the answers you have obtained. Your life is always the sum of all the choices you have made in the process. No matter what, life is a journey of self-discovery, a continual process of asking questions and seeking self-awakening answers from all the questions asked. The more questions you ask, the more powerful your thinking mind will become, and the more ready you will be to receive the self-intuitive answers.

The most important thing in questions-and-answers is to *experience* everything, not just to pursue the knowledge. As a matter of fact, knowledge can help, but it can also hinder. When you only follow what you *know*, and forget how and what you *feel*, you can easily be led down the wrong path. Extensive knowledge and even logical reasoning may not necessarily compound *true* human wisdom.

The bottom line: live every question you are going to ask yourself, and live in its full presence; be patient toward all those questions that you cannot find the answers right away. But true enlightenment may dawn on you one day when you find yourself asking fewer or even no more questions because by then you may already have got all the answers—*that* is the ultimate self-awakening.

Therefore, continue the process of self-reflecting all the questions you are going to ask yourself; without this self-reflection, you may continue to exist in the trauma of your *myasthenia gravis* diagnosis. Now, start asking questions to put yourself on the right path to intuiting the TAO of healing *myasthenia gravis*.

Asking all the questions *why* you have been afflicted with *myasthenia gravis* is your positive stepping backward into the past to fathom the ultimate truths of *why* you might have developed the devastating disease in the first place, thereby instrumental in moving you forward to healing the disease.

It is also important that you willingly *accept* your fate of getting the autoimmune disorder as the first step in your healing journey. It is futile to ask the question "Why *me*?", which is no more than a prolonged and negative stepping backward into the past with regret and remorse.

Embracing whatever that comes along in your life, no matter what, is life-transformation, which is one of the essentials of healing.

Acceptance and recognition of your current health conditions is your first positive step toward healing. Denial and despair, on the other hand, would only put more roadblocks on your healing journey.

Here are some of the questions you may like to ask to increase your knowledge:

What Is *Myasthenia Gravis*?

"*Myasthenia gravis*" is Latin and Greek in origin, which literally means "grave muscle weakness."

Myasthenia gravis is one of the many autoimmune diseases that afflict humans, and there are over one hundred of them.

What Is the Immune System?

> "In recent years science has learned that the human immune system is much more complicated than we thought."—**Dr. Philip F. Incao**, M.D.

First and foremost, you must have an understanding of your immune system in simple layman's terms:

- *Antibodies* are proteins that protect the human body from diseases and disorders, and they are like soldiers in an army.

- *Antigens* are foreign invaders in the form of bacteria and viruses that attack the human body.

- *T-cells*, a type of white blood cells originating from the bone marrow, either control and regulate the immune response or directly attack the infected cells.

The human immune system is complicated in that it affects the *whole* body system in many different ways. As such, it can heal but it can also harm you. It protects your cells and maintains your overall health through its production of antibodies (specific proteins) to help you fight against antigens (invaders to your body system). However, an impaired or dysfunctional immune system can adversely affect your overall health because it is the common denominator of more than one hundred autoimmune diseases.

The immune system is basically made up of four parts, and each part has its unique functions; it involves the whole human body, not just certain body organs and tissues. The complexity of the human immune system is a testament to the ingenuity and mystery of human creation.

The basic function of the immune system is to warn

the body of imminent dangers of viruses and bacteria (unfortunately, many of us just ignore these tale-telling signs, or simply fail to decipher these subtle body messages warning us of an imminent disease). In addition, the human immune system "remembers" these foreign invaders or antigens (the intention is to identify similar invaders in future for better disease-prevention purpose). Furthermore, the white blood cells in the immune system produce antibodies, which are chemicals that attach to and attack specific antigens. These white blood cells also send "messages" that will cause "inflammation" in response to an injury or antigen, and thus instrumental in preventing an infection from spreading elsewhere. In other words, they receive "chemical instructions" to nip the disease or the infection in the bud.

In short, the immune system serves different functions of *identification*, *activation*, *mobilization*, and *restoration*. It is akin to a police department in a city: it recognizes the city's potential crime scenario, takes strong measures to protect the public, trains the local police force to take appropriate actions, and regulates the law and order of the city.

What Are Autoimmune Diseases?

The occurrence of an autoimmune disease is a result of the breakdown or malfunction of the immune system. There are more than one hundred immune disorders and diseases.

The immune attack can target any area, such as the joints, causing rheumatoid arthritis, the thyroid gland, leading to an overactive or an underactive thyroid, and nerve cells, resulting in multiple sclerosis, among many others. Very often, the immune attack may have several targets; that is, if you have one autoimmune disease, you are also at risk for a second or even a third disease, especially if you have not taken good care of your immune system. In addition, an attack may have remission, followed by worsening of the symptoms. Therefore, the battle against an autoimmune disease is not only challenging, but also difficult and devastating.

Autoimmune diseases are becoming more rampant. By and large, women are more vulnerable to them than men are. Men have a higher incidence of mellitus diabetes and myocarditis (inflammation of the heart) than women; other than those, women are 3 to 6 times more prone to autoimmune diseases than their opposite sex.

Modern medicine is unable to explain or specifically identify some of the underlying causes of autoimmune diseases. Despite the advancement of modern science and technology, frustration and disappointment are part of modern medicine in the area of immune dysfunction. Without the capability to identify the exact causes of autoimmune diseases, there is no known cure to date. Accordingly, modern medicine focuses solely on addressing the symptoms rather than the causes.

What Are the Alternative Treatments?

In the past few decades, many have sought medical treatments for their "incurable" diseases, using herbs, detoxification, homeopathy, vitamins and minerals, among many others. This holistic non-drug approach to disease control and elimination has come to be known as alternative medicine.

Nowadays, medical universities in the United States, as well as in other parts of the world, are offering many alternative medicine courses and complementary medicine programs, while research studies on plant nutrients and vitamins and minerals are being conducted in university laboratories and clinical settings. They are all strong testaments to the effectiveness of alternative disease treatments.

Indeed, in this day and age, many people are becoming frustrated with conventional medicine's drugs, and the cut-and-burn approaches to disease. However, if you wish to seek an alternative approach to drug therapies, you must empower yourself with knowledge *before* you make any medical decision. But the decision should be totally *yours*, because nobody knows better than yourself the health conditions of your own body.

What Is the Prognosis of *Myasthenia Gravis*?

A prognosis is a prediction of the development of a disease, including whether the signs and symptoms will improve, worsen, or remain stable over time, as well as the expectation of the quality of life related to the development.

The prognosis of *myasthenia gravis* varies with different individuals. On the whole, symptoms may tend to worsen over longer periods of time, according to The Muscular Dystrophy Association. The muscular-weakness symptoms can fluctuate on a daily basis, with the most weakness in the evenings, especially after repeated muscle use.

TWO

THE WISDOM

What is "wisdom"? Is the word "wisdom" related to "philosophy"?

The word "philosophy" itself originally meant "the love of wisdom." Philosophy is *not* wisdom: it is just a concept of thinking, and a philosopher is merely a lover of that concept.

The Thinking Mind

Wisdom has much to do with the thinking mind: *how* it thinks.

The human brain is composed of grey matters and neurons that transmit information and messages; they are the building blocks of the brain for efficient functioning of the thinking mind.

Neurons are responsible for all human behaviors in the form of perceptions, which then trigger a mental process in the thinking mind that may result in an action or an emotion. If the process becomes instinctive, then the output in the form of actions or emotions is also automatic and predictable. That is how *attitudes* and *habits* are formed, including the fight-or-flight response to any given situation. This automatic or spontaneous mental process is often not "by choice" but by instinct.

But this so-called "learned" mental process is often responsible for the way you think and act, for your beliefs and emotions, for your actions or inactions, as well as for your overall choices and decisions resulting in your behaviors.

Therefore, it is important that: you *understand* how your thinking mind perceives and processes all your life experiences; you *recognize* your instinctive or automatic mental process; you *challenge* its reality or validity in order to see through the myth or even the deception; and you may then ultimately *change* your mental process by taking the appropriate actions accordingly.

The reality is that your thinking mind processes all your life experiences, and they then become your own thoughts and memories, which are the raw materials of your thinking process. They ultimately control and dominate your thinking mind.

In short, wisdom is the capability of the thinking mind to separate the sheep from the goats, that is, the truths from the untruths. To do just that, you have to understand *how* your thinking mind may be, affected, either positively or negatively, by your *life experiences*, by your *five senses*, and by your *subconscious mind*.

Your Life Experiences and Your Thinking Mind

Your experiences in life are the byproducts of what happens to you throughout your life journey, which is determined by two pivotal players: *choices* and *circumstances*.

- Choices result in actions or inactions, which often bring about consequences as well as circumstances that may affect your life in general and in specific.

- Circumstances are the events that happen to you and around you. There are two types: *self-inflicting internal circumstances*, such as your own procrastination, affecting all the subsequent events that happen in your life; *uncontrollable external circumstances*, such as accidents due to no fault of your own.

To illustrate, you had to complete a project and submit a report on that. You had sufficient time to do what you were supposed to do, but you made the *choice* to procrastinate until the last minute. An unforeseeable event took place and made it impossible for you to finish your work on time, and thus creating a self-inflicting *circumstance* of frustration and undue stress that might affect the other choices you subsequently had to make.

Personal choices may not be able to alter uncontrollable external circumstances, but they may still play a primary role in your *reactions* and *adaptations* to those external circumstances that are beyond your control.

To illustrate, in the devastating earthquake and tsunami that struck Japan in 2011, the Japanese people demonstrated their remarkable resilience in their reactions and subsequent adaptations to the uncontrollable external circumstances inflicted on them by nature.

Remember, your life is all about *choices* and *consequences*, and your living has much to do with *causes* and *results*—they may all become the components of your life experiences that may ultimately affect your health and the healing process of your *myasthenia gravis*.

Your Five Senses and Your Thinking Mind

The five senses form the basics of human sensations: sight, sound, smell, taste, and touch. But your five senses do not tell you *everything*; as a matter of fact, they may often give you only the half-truths.

The person who uses only the *vision* of his or her eyes is conditioned by what he or she sees. It is the *intuition* of the spirit that really perceives the reality. The wise have known for a long time that what we know through our eyes is not the same as the intuition of our spirit. If that is the case, sadly, most people rely only on what they see, thinking that "seeing is believing" and thus lose themselves in the realities of external things.

A case in point

In 1997, **Richard Alexander** from Indiana was convicted as a serial rapist because one of the victims and her fiancé insisted that he was the perpetrator based on what the victim and her fiancé claimed that "they *saw* with their own eyes."

But the convicted man was later exonerated and then subsequently released in 2001, based on new DNA science and other forensic evidence. Experts explained that a traumatic emotional experience, such as a rape, could "distort" the perception of an individual. That explains why the woman and her fiancé "swore" that Richard Alexander was the rapist, but evidently he was not.

Likewise, a traumatic experience, such as a *myasthenia gravis* diagnosis, may *distort* how you perceive your health and healing.

Your Subconscious Mind and Your Thinking Mind

Only your thinking mind can discern the truths from the delusions, the myths, or the half-truths. Only *you* have the answers to all the questions you ask about your own health and healing. To seek the truthful answers, you must also know *how* your conscious mind and your subconscious mind may work in your life.

The thinking mind—the consciousness of the brain—has two components: the *conscious* mind, and the *subconscious* mind. All your life experiences and perceptions of what happens to you processed by your five senses are stored in *both* your conscious mind and your subconscious mind.

Unlike your conscious mind, your subconscious mind embraces *indiscriminately* all your life experiences and perceptions of those happenings encountered in your life. Your subconscious mind is like the basement of your house, where you dump all the physical possessions you have been hoarding over the years.

Your conscious mind, on the other hand, is like the living area in your house, where you proudly display only some of the physical possessions that you may have chosen according to your likes and dislikes, such as a piece of antique furniture in the living room, or an original painting hanging on the wall in the dining room.

Your conscious mind *filters* all your thoughts—what you think is appropriate or relevant to your mental storage. In other words, your conscious mind *consciously* chooses what it wants to remember. Your subconscious mind, on the other hand, simply absorbs *all* your mental perceptions and reactions to *all* your experiences; it does not have the power to reason or to analyze any of your mental input. That is to say, it may not be able to tell the half-truths from the whole truths. Yet, it is your subconscious mind that *controls* your whole being, because your subconscious mind *dominates* your conscious mind. Yes, your conscious mind makes decisions, but it is your subconscious mind that directs and manipulates your conscious mind.

To illustrate, if you immediately turn on the TV as soon as you get home from work, most probably it is your subconscious mind telling your conscious mind that now is the time for relaxation and for watching the television. Likewise, many people talk on the cell phone while driving—that, too, is, their subconscious mind doing the driving, while their conscious mind is doing the talking.

Therefore, do not let your subconscious mind control and direct your conscious mind. Instead, learn to gain access to your subconscious mind through a *mental dialogue* in order to find out what is actually going on in your subconscious mind.

Meditation is an effective way of having a mental dialogue with the subconscious mind. Just like going through *everything* accumulated in your basement, you may find something valuable or totally trash to you; you may also find something that brings back good as well as bad memories. This internal mental dialogue of meditation with your subconscious mind may help you find out what is going on back there, and help you look more *objectively* and *non-judgmentally* at all the thoughts associated with your past experiences that have been stored in your subconscious mind over the years.

The Perspectives of Wisdom

There are different wise ways of seeing things in life, in the self, in others, and in the world around.

The Ancient Wisdom

With wisdom, the wise in the West began to seek answers to the many questions about the origin of man and the universe, as well as subsequently to those questions about the life and living of man. Western philosophy is generally said to begin in Greece, approximately five centuries before the birth of Jesus Christ.

Socrates

> "The only true wisdom is in knowing you know nothing."—**Socrates**

Socrates was one of the earliest Greek philosophers. He used his wisdom to explore and question many human things, including the good life, beauty, justice, and virtue.

Socrates was the first "positive psychologist" because he focused on the understanding of the human mind to find out the truths of many things.

Through a process of self-intuitive questioning, Socrates had transformed himself from an ignorant individual to one of the wisest of all men in his time. Like an empty cup, he was very open to receiving his all-empowering knowledge.

Plato

> "Wise men speak because they have something to say; fools because they have to say something."—**Plato**

Plato, a student of Socrates, examined the philosophical problems concerning the immortality of the soul, the benefits of being fair and just, the fact that evil is ignorance, and his groundbreaking Theory of Forms, which asserts that the physical world we are living in is not really the "real" world with ultimate reality existing beyond that physical world.

According to Plato, wisdom is using the mind to understand the moral reality in everyday life and living, which involves life choices and decisions.

Aristotle

> "Knowing yourself is the beginning of all wisdom."—**Aristotle**

Aristotle, another student of Socrates, was an artist, a scientist, a politician, and a philosopher.

For Aristotle, a thing is best understood by looking at its end, purpose, or goal. To illustrate, the goal of medicine is to achieve good health and wellness, and it is by seeing this ultimate goal that one best understands what medicine truly is.

The Eastern Wisdom

Around the time when Greek philosophy was emerging, the classic period of Chinese philosophy also flourished.

Confucius and Lao Tzu

> "The essence of knowledge is, having it, to apply it; not having it, to confess your own ignorance."—**Confucius**
>
> "Knowing others is intelligence.
> Knowing ourselves is true wisdom."
> —**Lao Tzu**

Confucius and Lao Tzu are two of the greatest thinkers throughout Chinese history. Confucius and Lao Tzu were contemporaries. According to legend, they met only once, disagreed, but respected each other's differing philosophies. Both of them have significantly dominated and impacted Chinese life and culture in a way unequaled by philosophies in the West.

Buddha

> "Change the way you look at things, and the things you look at will change."
> **—Buddha**

Buddha was an enlightened sage and teacher, who was born six centuries before the birth of Jesus Christ. He came from a royal family in the Himalayas, and had indulged himself in a world of luxury, until one day he witnessed three aspects of life that transformed him completely: the old, the sick, and the dying. Each of these experiences troubled him and made him question the meaning and transience of human life.

According to Buddha, the journey of human life begins with the understanding that human life is composed of pain and suffering—all caused by selfish cravings and personal desires. Detachment or letting go is the only path to overcoming the endless cycles of cravings and desires.

The Conventional Wisdom

> "Most people see what they expect to see, what they want to see, what they've been told to see, what conventional wisdom tells them to see—not what is right in front of them in its pristine condition."**—Vincent Bugliosi**

The conventional wisdom is "conventional" in the sense that the majority of people have already accepted it as the norm, with the explicit implication that others should also follow suit—something like a blueprint for all.

The conventional wisdom is mostly about compartmentalized and specialized knowledge. As an illustration, today's Western medicine has become so compartmentalized and specialized that holistic healing is often overlooked.

In addition, in the conventional wisdom, thinking is now becoming more logical and less reasonable. To illustrate, there are three virtues in the American culture: desire, efficiency, and punctuality for achievement. Paradoxically, they may become the three American vices, especially if there is too much emphasis on logic and not enough focus on the humanity side of reasoning. Desire, efficiency, and punctuality for achievement have often created undue stress for many in the American culture.

The conventional wisdom says that time is money. But time is not precious; time is but a construct. According to **Albert Einstein**, time is only relative. Efficiency and punctuality have imposed undue time-stress on nearly every one of us. Time-stress has led to multi-tasking. Nowadays, many of us are living for the future, and not in the present.

Given that it is human desire to see only one aspect of the truth we happen to perceive, we are more inclined to fashion it into a perfectly logical system, which we may also call the conventional wisdom. In short, the conventional wisdom is based on logic, rather than on imagination. Albert Einstein also has this to say: "Logic will get you from A to B. Imagination will take you everywhere."

If you really want to live an extraordinary life, you must think for yourself, do the unimagined, and create your own definition of the reality for living. In other words, you must live according to *your* own wisdom, and not just following the conventional wisdom, or that of someone else.

On the whole, the conventional wisdom lacks the element of true human wisdom, which is often found in the ancient wisdom. The conventional wisdom may have become for many the only roadmap to intelligent thinking.

The Spiritual Wisdom

> "Spiritual practice . . . involves, on the one hand, acting out of concern for others' well-being. On the other, it entails transforming ourselves so that we become more readily disposed to do so."
> **—Dalai Lama**

We are now living in a secular society, where science has become the dominant religion. As a result, nowadays, many people do not believe in the existence of God. His presence is no more than the presence of the sun, the moon, and the planets.

However, despite the absence of God in their lives, spirituality may still be present in the hearts of many.

Any human being living in the physical world has both a body, and a mind. This is an indisputable fact and reality. But do you *really* have a soul?

If you do not *totally live* in your body, you *do* have a soul or spirit. If you do not *totally focus* on yourself all the time, you may then also have a glimpse of your soul or spirit.

If you believe in God, your soul is your spiritual *connection* and *communication* with Him in the form of your daily prayers, moments of self-awakening, and occasional divine guidance and inspiration from Him.

If you do not have a specific religion, but still believe in the control of a Being greater than yourself, your soul or spirit is your *understanding* of the unexplainable control and the natural cycle of all things—that is, certain things in life happen without any rhyme or reason, which are completely beyond human control, and certain things always follow a natural cycle, such as life is followed by death.

If you are a non-believer, but still a decent human being, your soul or spirit is your *conscience*, which intuitively tells you what is right and wrong, and not just following the law and order of your country.

Therefore, in different ways, we may *all* have a soul or spirit, although some of us may either consciously or unconsciously separate ourselves from it. The soul or spirit is just like a shadow of ourselves: sometimes we see more of it, and other times we see less of it, but it is always following us wherever we go, whether we like it or not.

Believing in spirituality may give you the miracle of *becoming* and *transforming*, which is spiritual wisdom to make you become a better and a healthier individual.

So, believing in spirituality may enhance your consciousness of your own true self with the deep desire to become wholesome again. If you have been diagnosed with *myasthenia gravis*, you may begin to sense your incompleteness and your own inadequacy in your struggle against the disease. You may then begin to turn to someone or something that can truly change and transform you into a better being with better health.

Change is external, but transformation is internal. Change requires you to look outside of you; transformation comes from looking inside of you. Change may have a negative connotation in that you want to get rid of something undesirable in order to receive something desirable.

Transformation is enhancement of something which in itself is good, and which is already innate in you. Transformation is rediscovery of what is already there inside you, but has somehow become invisible to your naked eyes, imperceptible to your mind, and unintelligible to your soul, due to their misalignment. Transformation is often the path to enlightenment, which is self-awakening to true wisdom.

In short, spiritual wisdom is an awareness of the true self with the desire to become wholesome, connecting the body and the spirit through the mind.

Remember, the mind dominates both the body and the soul. Even if you are a dedicated and devoted believer of God, it is your mind, and not your soul, that dominates your whole being. Why? It is because your soul is just an advisor or a consultant. Therefore, it is all up to your mind whether or not to take the initiative to seek the advice, as well as whether or not to make the final decision to act and react according to the advice or instruction given. So, compared to the mind, the soul plays only a secondary role.

Having said that, it does not mean that the soul or spirit does not play a pivotal role in the body-mind-soul inter-connection. As a matter of fact, your soul is the source of life force in the form of invisible energy to your body and your mind to give them direction and supervision in the physical world.

The truth of the matter is that humans are given a physical body, a mind, and a soul or spirit. The body, living in the material world, is equipped with the five senses to live and survive in the physical environment. The mind, as the mediator between the body and the soul, is given the gift of free will, which is the freedom to process any input in the form of thoughts and inspirations from both the body and the soul. That is, whenever we wish to do something, the soul intuitively provides the instinctive advice and judgment, the mind then gives the analysis and the interpretation, and the body eventually executes the appropriate action or decision of the mind. Therefore, the human mind plays a pivotal role in the understanding and the interpretation of some of these ultimate truths in human existence.

The Essence of True Wisdom

True wisdom is much more than knowledge or intelligence. It has much to do with the processing of information by the thinking mind. It requires much clarity and concentration of the thinking mind to see things as they really are, and not as what they are meant or supposed to be. Accordingly, being knowledgeable may suggest smartness but not necessarily the true wisdom of an individual. After all, humans are all limited in their capacity and capability to acquire knowledge, which is often unlimited. Therefore, to use what is limited for the unlimited is irrational. True wisdom, on the other hand, is empowering the thinking, which is potentially unlimited, to apply the limited knowledge acquired to understand the true nature of the self, of others, and of the world around—which is unlimited.

True wisdom is innate and inside you, but you just have to *look inside* you, just as **Eckhart Tolle** says in the beginning of his book **The Power of Now**:

> "A beggar has been sitting by the side of a road for over thirty years. One day a stranger walked by. 'Spare some change?' mumbled the beggar, mechanically holding out his old baseball cap. 'I have nothing to give you,' said the stranger. Then he asked: 'What's that you are sitting on?' 'Nothing,' replied the beggar. 'Just an old box. I have been sitting on it for as long as I can remember.' 'Ever looked inside?' asked the stranger. 'No,' said the beggar. 'What's the point? There's nothing in there.' 'Have a look inside,' insisted the stranger. The beggar managed to prey open the lid. With astonishment, disbelief, and elation, he saw that the box was filled with gold."

Yes, *looking inside* is the key to attaining and understanding true human wisdom. When you look more deeply within yourself, you may become awakened and even enlightened.

Self-wakening is an understanding of who you really are, and not who you wish you were, based on the thoughts of your thinking mind.

Your Thoughts Make You Who You Are

Descartes, the great French philosopher, made his famous statement: "I think, therefore I am." That means, you think, and your thoughts then become who and what you *think* you are. But that may not be the *real* you.

You are who you are by virtue of your *thinking*, and your thoughts then become your personality.

You are the products of your thoughts, because you *identify* yourself with all the thoughts in your subconscious mind. In other words, you "think" you are who you are by reason of the thoughts absorbed and stored in your subconscious mind. Because their absorption is automatic and spontaneous, your subconscious mind is incapable of analyzing or validating their authenticity.

Self-awakening is your realization that your mind power is totally within your control. What you really need is self-discovery through self-analysis with complete honesty. If you learn to *observe*, *control*, and *change* your thoughts, you will then become the master of your thinking mind, thereby instrumental in transforming who you *think* you are and what you have now become into your *true* self.

Your Thoughts Put You Where You Are

You are where you are right now by choice and not by chance. That is, the onset of *myasthenia gravis* is your choice. You may not like where you are, but you will continue to remain there unless you are willing to *change* your thinking mind and to accept the notion that you are where you are for the specific purpose of learning *how* to grow and transform yourself so that you may get away from where you are right now—that is, experiencing the symptoms of *myasthenia gravis*. Without that acute awareness, you will continue to remain in your status quo, that is, being unhealed of *myasthenia gravis*.

Remember, your circumstances do not make you the person you are; they only *reflect* what you *truly* are. So, if you do not like what you have now become due to the circumstances, you must be prepared to *transform* yourself by changing your thinking mind. You are the creator of your own conditions and circumstances.

An instructor In a motorcycle training course once said, "If you're confronted by an imminent obstacle, don't fixate on it, or else you'll steer right into it. Instead, look above and past it to where you need to go, in order to avoid it."

Likewise, focusing on your problematic conditions and undesirable circumstances related to your *myasthenia gravis* will make you not only head toward them but also continue to remain in them.

The bottom line: true wisdom—whether it is the ancient wisdom, the conventional wisdom, or the spiritual wisdom—is knowing the truths about yourself, as well as about others and the world around you that might have contributed to your current affliction of *myasthenia gravis*.

THREE

THE TAO

Healing begins with the mind, and not with the body. But the mind can both heal and harm. Therefore, wisdom plays a critical role in the healing process—more specifically, the TAO wisdom of **Lao Tzu**.

What exactly is the TAO?

The TAO is the wisdom of Lao Tzu, the ancient sage from China. who was born with grey hair (a sign of wisdom related to old age and experience). He was well known for his profound wisdom, despite the fact that he did not have any disciples or followers, like many ancient sages did.

According to legend, Lao Tzu was just about to leave China for Tibet, because at that time China was a war zone with many warlords fighting one another. At the city gate, riding backward on an ox, he was detained and was told that he could not leave the country unless he had put down in writing all his brilliant ideas on human wisdom. Reluctantly and defiantly, he put down his profound wisdom in only 5,000 words. That was how *Tao Te Ching* came into existence.

The TAO Essentials

Despite its apparent mysticism and paradoxical nature, the TAO is not difficult to understand. All you need is an empty mindset with *reverse* thinking, which is very different from the conventional way of pre-conditioned thinking.

There was the well-known story of a professor visiting a Zen master and seeking information about Zen (an ancient Asian philosophy evolved from the TAO). The Zen master kept pouring tea into the already filled-up teacup in the professor's hand, while the professor continued his own non-stop talking. The moral of the story: you must keep an empty mind before you can be open and receptive to any new idea; having a pre-conditioned mindset is a common characteristic of the contemporary human mind.

According to Lao Tzu, the essentials of TAO cannot be expressed in words. TAO is not a concept. TAO is something that existed before there were words, before there was human speech, before there was even thought. TAO is something that must be *lived* and *experienced* in order to fully appreciate what it is. As a matter of fact, words in themselves are not important because they are not the truths. They do not teach; they only *point* to the truths, which have to be self-intuited. There is a saying: "The teacher and the taught together create the teaching." That is to say, teaching is the embodiment of *awareness*, *assimilation*, and *application* of understanding, without which there is no learning or teaching, not to mention true wisdom. In other words, the TAO is all about your own *understanding* of the self, of others, and of all the things around the self. But nobody can *make* you understand—not even words—and only your own *thinking mind* can.

Humility and the Ego-Self

If the TAO can be expressed in one word, that word is "humility."

So, what is meant by "humility"?

The opposite of "humility" is "pride", which inflates the ego-self.

Then, what is the ego-self?

The ego-self is the "false" identity that an individual has created for himself or herself based on the thoughts stored in the subconscious mind as memories and expectations. Because thoughts of memories existed only in the past, and thoughts of expectations will exist only in the future, therefore, they do not really exist in the present, and thus are unreal.

Without your ego-self, you may then see your true self, as well as the truths of anything and everything about you and around you. Your ego-self is your self-deceptive perceptions of who you think you are, based on years of your own self-illusions.

Only humility can make you see your true identity, that is, who you *really* are, and not who you wish you were. Humility can be attained only by living a simple lifestyle, and by letting go of all your attachments that erroneously define who you think you are. Remember, you are living in the physical world with all the trimmings of your life that are not easy to let go of. and that is why you need profound human wisdom, in particular, that of the TAO.

According to the TAO, humility has to do with the *self*, which has to do with the mind, which has to do with the thinking process, and which has to do with human thoughts. They all have to do with how you *perceive* your own life experiences, as well as how your *process* your thoughts on those perceptions.

But *how* can humility heal?

Without knowing your true self, you do not have wisdom. Without wisdom, you do not know how to seek knowledge. Without *true* wisdom. you do not know how to *apply* the knowledge acquired to heal yourself.

No Fear and No Expectation

Human fear comes in different forms: instinctive fear, such as fear of a dangerous environment; and psychological fear, such as anxiety, paranoia, and worry. The former is more natural and grounded than the latter, which is based more on the factor "might." But all fear has to do with failure to do something, and ultimately death. Once you have illusively identified yourself with that fear in your mind, the fear begins to overtake you as a person, and you then become the very thing you are afraid of.

Consumed with fear, your mind then begins to *expect* something different from what you fear. Any expectation will project the thinking mind into the future; that is, you begin to live in the future, as opposed to living in the present. But the future is uncertain and unreal. The more you project your thinking mind into the future as expectations, the more self-delusions you have created to distort your thinking.

But with no fear, there is no expectation, and with no expectation, your mind remains in the now.

No Judgment and No Pain

Anticipation comes with expectation. To have your expectation fulfilled, your mind then begins its judgment—picking and choosing what you think may fulfill your expectation.

But judgment often comes with a hefty price: pain. Human life is never pain-free or sorrow-free. Failures and frustrations—they all originate from expectations unfulfilled—often lead to human pain and stress.

Fear of human pain only intensifies your mind to pick and choose: picking what you think will help you avoid the imaginary pain; and choosing what you think will help you fulfill your expectation. In the process of choosing and judging, you often make mistakes and wrong choices, and thus creating only more fear and more pain, as well as leading to vicious circles of expectations and frustrations due to unfulfilment.

No Control and No Over-Doing

According to the TAO, anything and everything in this world follow a natural cycle of spontaneity: what goes up must also come down. Therefore, all these extremes in human experiences are not only temporary but also unnatural; they are just the pendulum swinging back and forth from one end to the other.

Accordingly, it is human folly to attempt any control to avoid or resist experiencing these natural swings. By doing so, man throws himself out of balance with nature, and thus not only intensifies but also unduly prolongs his pains and sufferings.

The bottom line: do not control what is beyond human control; instead, just accept and embrace the uncontrollable.

The TAO emphasizes "wu-wei" (無為): "Wu" (無)

means "no" and "wei" (為) means "doing." Due to the literal translation of the original text, "wu-wei" is often misinterpreted as "non-doing," and therefore even regarded as a "passive" way of looking at life by Lao Tzu. "Under-doing" or "nothingness" is a more appropriate translation of "wu-wei."

According to the TAO, you should do what needs to be done—no more and no less.

There is a Chinese idiom that says: "Push the boat with the current." It means the wisdom of availing an opportunity to move forward but without exerting any extra effort. It is the wisdom of the choice to empty oneself and then go with the flow of the current, instead of against it. "Non-doing" is an act of spontaneity and effortlessness in accomplishing all things.

There was a Chinese story . . . 畫蛇添足 about a competition in drawing, in which candidates were asked to draw a snake in detail. One of the candidates finished his drawing sooner than all the rest of the competitors. Thinking that extra effort might give him extra credit, he took it upon himself to add some legs with fine details to the snake. As a result of his extra effort, instead of his "non-doing," he was disqualified and lost the competition.

Living in the Present and Letting Go

Given that the human mind is addicted to thinking thoughts in the past or projecting them into the future, and that these thoughts thus create the false ego-self, the present moment holds the key to understanding the *real* self of an individual.

According to the TAO, only the present is real: the past was already gone, and the future, uncertain and unpredictable, is yet to come. When the mind stays in the present, it has clarity of thinking that does not see the ego-self. But when the mind constantly alternates between the past and the future, it then becomes self-deceptive and self-delusional, and thus creating and sustaining the false ego-self with unreal expectations, requiring wrong choices followed by over-doing—they all lead to human miseries and sufferings.

In the present moment, you can *objectively* and *non-judgmentally* observe both your past thoughts and their future projections, and thus you can effectively *validate* them for their veracity.

If your thoughts are false, distracting, misleading, and unreal, just detach yourself from them. Letting go of all attachments is the way to humility.

The bottom line: with humility, you may then begin your journey of the TAO of healing *myasthenia gravis*.

FOUR

THE JOURNEY

One of **Lao Tzu**'s famous sayings is "A journey of a thousand miles begins with the first step." The TAO journey of healing *myasthenia gravis* is a great undertaking: every step is as important as the first; and each step is as firm as the previous one. The Chinese often like to say "feet stepping on solid and steady ground." Your healing journey is the sum of all the steps you are going to take.

Before you take your first step, ponder on this reality: in life, all humans have two desires or pursuits—happiness and healthiness, which not only often come with many delusions and illusions but also always are unattainable and unsustainable. But the TAO may give you self-intuition and self-enlightenment to help you along your own journey of healing *myasthenia gravis*.

The Step of No Desire and No Intent

It is *your* journey, and only *you* can take *your* first step. So, you must *choose* to take your first step to go on that healing journey.

To continue on your journey, paradoxically, you must show no desire to heal and no intent to reach your destination.

But why?

The desire for good health may be difficult to sustain for someone who is currently confronted with the many health issues related to *myasthenia gravis*. It may seem not only difficult but almost impossible for that individual to restore natural health and get well again. Worse, ill health may even make that individual feel depressed and forget to take care of the body, and thus allowing the body's malfunctions to continue and deteriorate further.

A wise traveler on a long journey has no fixed plans, and is not intent upon arriving the destination within a certain time frame. But that traveler is ready to use all the situations and all the people encountered to help him along the long journey.

Likewise, healing is a long, on-going process, and not a destination. With innate and inexplicable power, it may appear that everyone and everything along your journey are also playing a part in facilitating in your favor all your endeavors in healing your *myasthenia gravis*.

The bottom line: take your first step of no desire and no intent for healing so as to change and to overcome any attitude of confusion and even despair related to the trauma of your *myasthenia gravis* diagnosis. On your healing journey, with no intent upon arriving at the destination any time soon, you will continue to keep yourself moving forward, and you will then go the long distance on your long healing journey.

The TAO

According to the TAO, being free of desires is your path to detachment, and thus giving you clarity of thinking to start your own healing journey.

Paradoxically, if you have no desire to desire for change or healing, there is *stillness*, in which you may see yourself gradually changing for the better in order to slowly heal yourself:

> "To live a life of harmony, we need letting life live by itself. . .
>
> So, follow the Way.
> Stop striving to change ourselves: we are naturally changing."
> (Lao Tzu, **Tao Te Ching**, Chapter 57)
>
> "Accordingly, we do not rush into things.
> We neither strain nor stress.
> We let go of success and failure.
> We patiently take the next necessary step, a small step and one step at a time.
> We relinquish our conditioned thinking. Being our true nature, we help all beings

return to their own nature too."
(Lao Tzu, ***Tao Te Ching***, Chapter 64)

According to the TAO, a good traveler neither has fixed plans, nor shows any effort to arrive at the destination:

> "The softest thing in the world
> overcomes what seems to be the hardest.
>
> That which has no form
> penetrates what seems to be impenetrable.
>
> That is why we exert effortless effort.
> We act without over-doing.
> We teach without arguing.
>
> This is the Way to true wisdom.
> This is not a popular way
> because people prefer over-doing."
> (Lao Tzu, ***Tao Te Ching***, Chapter 43)

Begin your healing journey, and take your first step with effortless effort and humble simplicity:

> "Those, who think they know, know not the Way.
> Those, who think they know not, find the Way.
>
> Simplicity is clarity.
> It is a blessing to learn from those
> with humble simplicity.
> Those with an empty mind

will learn to find the Way.
The Way reveals the secrets of the universe:
the mysteries of the realm of creation;
the manifestations of all things created.
The essence of the Way is to show us
how to live in fullness and return to our origin."
(Lao Tzu, **Tao Te Ching**, Chapter 65)

The Step of Awareness and Mindfulness

On your healing journey, you must always be aware of your steps and mindful of your surrounding.

Awareness

Awareness is deep concentration of the mind to know what is happening to the body. This is essential to healing of the body. Nobody—not even your doctor—knows your body better than yourself, but you have to be *aware* of it.

Breathing is your awareness of what is happening to your body. It is critically important to your overall health. Breathing gives life. Without food and water, you may still survive for a while, but without your breath, you die within minutes.

Breathing has to do with the lungs, which serve two main functions: to get life-giving oxygen from the air into the body, and to remove toxic carbon dioxide from the body. So, do not compromise your lung functions with nicotine or any drug.

Breathing patterns are critical to health. That is, *how* you breathe may positively or negatively affect your body organs and hormones. For example, taking short, shallow breaths, you are in fact telling your brain that a threat exists, which then stimulates a stress response, and thus creating destructive thinking patterns in your brain. Conversely, taking long and deep breaths, you are sending positive signals to your brain for positive thinking patterns. When you own your breath, you have calm and peace. Breathing is just a simple strategy for instant stress-relief.

Diaphragm breathing

Learn how to breathe right: diaphragm breathing is natural breathing; it is the *complete* breath.

Consciously change your breathing patterns. Use your diaphragm to breathe (the diaphragm muscle separating your chest from your abdomen). Place one hand on your breastbone, feeling that it is raised, and put the other hand above your waist, feeling the diaphragm muscle moving up and down. Deep breathing with your diaphragm gives you complete breath. This is how you do diaphragm breathing:

- Sit comfortably.

- Begin your slow exhalation through your nose.

- Contract your abdomen to empty your lungs.

- Begin your slow inhalation and simultaneously make your belly bulge out.

- Continuing your slow inhalation, now, slightly contract your abdomen and simultaneously lift your chest and hold.

- Continue your slow inhalation, and slowly raise your shoulders. This allows the air to enter fully into your lungs to attain the complete breath.

- Retain your breath and slightly raise your shoulders for a count of 5.

- Very slowly exhale the air. Your upper chest deflates first, and then your abdomen relaxes in.

- Repeat the process.

Learn to slowly prolong your breath, especially your exhalation. Relax your chest and diaphragm muscle, so that you can extend your exhalation, making your breathing out longer and complete. To prolong your exhalation, count "one-and-two-and-three" as you breathe in and breathe out. Make sure that they become balanced. Once you have mastered that, then try to make your breathing out a little longer than your breathing in.

Practice diaphragm breathing until it becomes

second nature to you. Diaphragm breathing is relaxing and stress-relieving.

Alternate-nostril breathing

Alternate-nostril breathing is a basic Yoga breathing exercise to balance the right side and the left side of your brain. This exercise is especially ideal for enhancing your body balance (critically important, especially if you may have double vision), as well as internal harmony and stress-relief.

The left side of your brain governs the right side of your body, including your speech and logical thinking, while the right side of your brain governs the left side of your body, including your creativity and intuition. Achieving balance and harmony between the two sides of your brain is critical to mind healing for deep relaxation and stress-relief. You can balance your mental energy from the right and the left side of the brain while practicing your alternate-nostril breathing during meditation or a mind-relaxation session. Practice alternate-nostril breathing everyday for stress-relief.

This is how to practice alternate-nostril breathing:

- Place your thumb and ring finger lightly on your right and your left nostrils, respectively, with your index and middle fingers resting lightly on your forehead just between your eyebrows.

- Exhale deeply through BOTH nostrils.

- Press your thumb against the RIGHT nostril to CLOSE it.

- Breathe in through your LEFT nostril. Count 8.

- CLOSE your LEFT nostril by pressing down your ring finger. Now, BOTH nostrils are closed. Retain the air, and count 4.

- OPEN your RIGHT nostril, and breathe out. Count 8.

- With the LEFT nostril still CLOSED, breathe in through the RIGHT nostril. Count 8.

- CLOSE the RIGHT nostril. Now, BOTH nostrils are closed. Retain the air, and count 4.

- OPEN the LEFT nostril, and breathe out with the RIGHT nostril still closed. Count 8.

- With the RIGHT nostril closed, you have breathed out through the LEFT nostril; you have now completed one round of the breathing exercise.

- Begin the second round by breathing in through the LEFT nostril, and repeat the above.

Here is a short summary of alternative-nostril breathing:

- Breathe out through BOTH nostrils.

- Breathe in through the LEFT nostril (count 8).

- Close BOTH nostrils, and retain the air (count 4).

- Breathe out through the RIGHT nostril (count 8).

- Breathe in through the RIGHT nostril (count 8).

- Close BOTH nostrils, and retain the air (count 4).

- Breathe out through the LEFT nostril (count 8).

- Breathe in through the LEFT nostril and repeat the whole process.

Practice your alternate-nostril breathing to create your acute awareness and concentration, as well as to enhance your internal body balance to de-stress yourself.

Mindfulness

Mindfulness is acute mental awareness, which is deep concentration of the body and the mind for their inter-connection: the body is created to support the mind. To sharpen your mind power, you must enhance the awareness of your body *first*. If you feel that your body, mind, and soul are not connected, most probably there is lack of body awareness by the mind in the first place. Therefore, mindfulness begins with awareness of the body first.

Most of us do not pay much attention to the body—except when we experience physical pain—let alone paying attention to the mind. But mental attention is important to the wisdom in stress-free living. The mind and the body are inter-connected. Your mental attention is essentially your body consciousness, or your attention to the physical conditions and the needs of your body in relation to how your mind thinks. Understanding this intricate relationship may help you relax both your body and your mind.

Are you always paying conscious attention to your body at all times?

The way you normally eat speaks volumes of the degree or intensity of your body awareness. It is not the food you eat, but *how* you are eating your food that shows your body awareness. While eating, if you are reading your newspaper, watching your TV, working on your computer, or checking your cell phone, you are *not* paying *any* attention to your body, which at that very moment is supposed to be *eating* and not doing multitasking.

Train your mind to pay more attention to *how* your body reacts when you are eating, such as chewing your food thoroughly, slowing down your eating process by tasting each morsel of the food in your mouth. Always give the full presence of your mind to your meal. Again, how often you look at something without seeing it at all because your mind is not paying its full attention to what you are looking at. When your mind is not paying its full attention, your body becomes incapacitated; only when your body becomes fully conscious, then your mental capacity will then become enhanced and sharpened. Body awareness is simply paying full attention to what your body is doing at that present moment. In other words, be more conscious of what your body is doing when you are eating, walking, or doing anything routine. In any life situation, even while doing your dishes, you can use your total body awareness to switch off your thinking mind, and give it a meaningful break for your stress-relief.

The bottom line: with awareness and mindfulness, you may then begin to see the ultimate truths in anything and everything—including who you really are, all those close and related to you, as well as what is happening to and around you, including your *myasthenia gravis*.

The TAO

Awareness is knowing who you really are, instead of who you wish you were. This is the only path to humility, which gives you an empty mindset with reverse thinking to *rethink* what is already in your pre-conditioned mind:

> "Can we embrace both good fortunes and misfortunes in life?
> Can we breathe as easily as innocent babies?
> Can we see the world created as it is without judgment?
> Can we accept both the desirable and the undesirable?
> Can we express compassion to all without being boastful?
> Can we watch the comings and goings of things without being perturbed?
>
> Saying "yes" to all of the above is spiritual wisdom from the Creator,
> who watches the comings and goings in the world He created."
> (Lao Tzu, **Tao Te Ching**, Chapter 10)

According to the TAO, awareness is:

> "watchful, like a man crossing a winter stream;
> alert, like a man aware of danger;
> courteous, like a visiting guest;
> yielding, like ice about to melt;
> simple, like a piece of uncarved wood;
> hollow, like a cave;
> opaque, like muddy water."
> (Lao Tzu, **Tao Te Ching**, Chapter 15)

Awareness may also awaken you to the many

differences in your own perceptions of *myasthenia gravis*:

> "In the absence of the Creator, we forget who we really are.
> Then we turn to other things to define who we are, what is good and moral.
>
> In the presence of the Creator, we act according to our hearts,
> instead of relying on rules and regulations from those above us.
>
> Rules and regulations may bring fairness and justice,
> but no more than a pretense of life.
> A pretense of life is our inability to love indiscriminately.
> Then we insist on those above us to heal our suffering,
> which originates from ourselves."
> (Lao Tzu, **Tao Te Ching**, Chapter 18)

Mindfulness is the deep understanding of your body: *how* and *why* you are sick. The reason why a sage is not ill is that he sees illness as illness, and not as something else:

> "Not knowing the Way,
> but pretending we know,
> we remain ignorant, and suffer.
>
> Knowing that we do not know,

we pursue its wisdom:
knowing its origin,
knowing its ending,
and knowing our true nature."
(Lao Tzu, **Tao Te Ching**, Chapter 71)

Mindfulness is watching and observing what is happening to your body, as well as anything and everything around you:

> "The Creator seems elusive amid the changes of life.
> At times, He seems to have forsaken His creations.
> In reality, He is simply observing the comings and goings of their follies.
>
> Likewise, we watch the comings and goings of our likes and dislikes, of our desires and fears.
> But we do not identify with them.
> With no judgment and no preference,
> we see the mysteries of creation."
> (Lao Tzu, **Tao Te Ching**, Chapter 7)

With mindfulness, you become a watcher and an observer, leading to the rebirth and renewal of your thinking mind:

> "The Creator has no judgment, no preference:
> He treats everything and everyone alike.
> Every manifestation attests to the mysteries of His creation.

So, we, too, embrace everything and everyone with no judgment, no preference.
His grace, never depleting and forever replenishing, shows us the Way.
Judgment and preference separate us from His grace, causing attachment.
Only with His grace do we find renewal and rebirth along the Way."
(Lao Tzu, **Tao Te Ching**, Chapter 5)

With awareness and mindfulness, you may attain the true wisdom of knowing yourself:

"Knowing others is intelligence.
Knowing ourselves is true wisdom.
Overcoming others is strength.
Overcoming ourselves is true power.

Understanding that we have everything we need,
we count our blessings.
Identifying with our own true nature,
we hold fast to what endures."
(Lao Tzu, **Tao Te Ching**, Chapter 33)

Awareness and emptiness provide you with an empty mindset to take your next step of unlearning and relearning everything related to healing your *myasthenia gravis*.

The Step of Unlearning and Relearning

Your healing journey requires a compass and a roadmap: the former to show you the direction of your journey; the latter to tell you where you are right now.

To heal, you must *unlearn* what you have previously learned, that is, letting go of all your preconceptions related to all the *hows* and the *whys* you might have got your *myasthenia gravis* in the first place. Remember, the knowledge you are currently having may have been generated by the limited and the finite material world you are living in.

Life itself is a sacred journey involving change, growth, and self-discovery. Knowledge is self-empowering, but it has to be distilled by true human wisdom. Therefore, to deepen your love of heath and your quest for health and healing, you must seek not just knowledge but also wisdom in order to expand your vision and stretch your soul so that you may stay both physically healthy and spiritually wise. Your knowledge and wisdom may provide you with meaning and direction to continue with every step of your long healing journey.

Unlearning Pharmaceutical Drugs

As we age, our self-made energy from the food we have consumed over the years begins to decline, and this is evidenced by our inability or difficulty to cope with the stressors of life. These stressors may have come in many different forms, such as overexposure to sunlight, polluted air, contaminated water, and a host of other lifestyle factors of modern life. After decades of abuse to our bodies, our choices—whether we have made them knowingly, or they have been imposed unwittingly on ourselves—begin to take their toll, resulting in the development of chronic conditions and degenerative diseases. To add insult to injury, our metabolic slowdown that comes with the natural process of aging makes it even more difficult to maintain our health and energy.

To deal with our health issues, many of us may desire a quick-fix, and thus turn to pharmaceutical drugs, which are toxic chemicals that only address the symptoms but without removing the causes of the health conditions.

Unfortunately, unsafe and toxic pharmaceutical drugs are prevalent. This is an indisputable fact! Unreliable drug tests abound in the medical and pharmaceutical research communities. Drug tests prior to their FDA approval may not be reliable due to the following reasons:

- Pharmaceutical companies may often influence medical researchers, through coercion, incentive, and even threat, to produce the desired results in clinical trials. There have been many cases of data fabrication in clinical trials of drugs in order to facilitate their intended applications.

- Clinical trials usually involve a small number of people, and may not truly reflect the outcome of those who will ultimately be using those drugs after their approval by FDA.

- Drugs tested on animal models may be biased and even irrelevant. An artificially-induced disease in non-human animals may not yield results relevant to a spontaneous, naturally-occurring human disease.

Relearning Pharmaceutical Drugs

Regularly taking pharmaceutical drugs does not make you live longer because longevity is always drug-free. This makes sense: taking too many pharmaceutical drugs means your body is already stressed by many physical ailments. Ironically, these drugs may do a further disservice to you by ingesting more toxins into your already toxic body.

Pharmaceutical drugs do not heal a disease; they only temporarily suppress the disease symptoms. Remember, when you give your body a drug to replace a substance that your body is capable of making itself, you body then becomes weaker and will begin not only to manufacture less of that substance, but also to become more dependent on the outside source, which is usually the drug itself. Over time, you will become no longer drug-free.

Unfortunately, no drug can give you insight into the circumstance that created your problems in the first place. At best, it can only temporarily assuage the physical pain created by your situation. Remember, there are no miracle drugs—only wholesome natural self-healing. Utilize your body's natural self-healing power, rather than relying on those unsafe pharmaceutical drugs. Keep yourself drug-free as much as and as long as possible!

However, it does not imply that you must desist from taking your medications prescribed by your doctor. Rather, it suggests you should always be more alert to the side effects of the drugs you are currently taking; you should not readily reach out for unsafe pharmaceutical drugs, especially over-the-counter ones, without any second thought as if they were coupons or silver bullets.

Unlearning Conventional Medicine

First of all, conventional or Western medicine is never drug-free: it is based on the medical model in which a doctor identifies a set of symptoms of a patient and makes a diagnosis to confirm the doctor's examination. An approved treatment for that diagnosis is then applied to the patient. Commonly, the treatment may be a chemical one in the form of a pharmaceutical drug to interfere with the natural healing mechanism in the patient's own body with the express purpose of removing those undesirable symptoms. The patient, too eager to be relieved of the symptoms, often readily concurs to the application of those unsafe pharmaceutical drugs.

Sadly, such intellectual process of cure does not take into account the patient's individual physical, mental, and spiritual problems, which may be the fundamental causes of that disease in the first place.

In addition, conventional medicine does not take into consideration the basic health concept that your body is designed to regulate and repair itself, and therefore does not address natural healing, which is always made in deference to the more invasive procedures, such as administering a drug, which only infuse your body with more toxins.

Relearning Unconventional Medicines

Learn many other unconventional medicines that may provide you with many other alternative healings that are not only natural but also less invasive.

Ayurveda Medicine

Ayurveda medicine is based on 5,000 years of the expertise and knowledge of sages with respect to health and self-healing. It is the oldest self-healing system in existence; as a matter of fact, it is the first world medicine. Originally, there were two schools of Ayurveda: the school of physicians and the school of surgeons. Through many centuries of transformation, they have now evolved into a scientifically veritable and classifiable medical system, a widely used system of self-healing in India.

The essence of Ayurveda wisdom is self-discovery and self-growth; they make you realize that many answers to health and wellness are all within yourself.

Aromatherapy

Aromatherapy, another ancient self-healing art, uses essential oils to promote health and wellness of the skin, the body, the mind, and the soul for complete and holistic self-healing. The aroma, from the essential oils of certain plants through the bursting of their tiny glands, has therapeutic self-healing effects. These plants, having accumulated the radiant energy from the sun, produce essential oils that have anti-fungal and anti-inflammatory self-healing properties.

Ancient healers were holistic: to them, self-healing was a transcendent art. They believed in the self-healing power of plant energy; accordingly, if plants could heal the body with their energies, they could also heal the mind too, given that the body and the mind were but one. Based on this belief, ointments, oils, incenses, infusions, and poultices were widely used in ancient healing in China, India, Greece, Babylon, and Egypt.

Naturopathy

Naturopathy, or naturopathic medicine, is an integrated system of primary health care based on the use of herbs and foods for medicine, exposure to fresh air and sunlight, and hydrotherapy (the use of hot and cold water application), such as steam or sauna, to enhance wellness for purpose of self-healing.

Naturopathy is based on the philosophy that all living things have an innate ability to heal themselves due to an innate vital force that promotes self-cleansing, self-repair, and therefore self-healing. The key to self-healing is to address the depressed immune system, the disruptive hormonal changes, the disorderly nervous and the dysfunctional elimination systems. Once balance is restored, then the body will begin its self-healing, although it may be a long and slow process. Given that it focuses on the causes of diseases, rather than just on the treatment of their symptoms, naturopathy is holistic medicine.

Chinese Medicine

Self-healing begins with the mind, which can generate energy to accomplish the task of healing. Self-healing is energy healing.

According to the laws of physics, there is energy in everything, and everything gives out invisible energy, including the sun, the moon, and the human body. As a matter of fact, everything is some form of energy, which is either positive or negative. For example, your thinking, too, involves energy, without which the mind cannot function. If you "think" you can heal yourself, your mind sends out positive energy to your body for self-healing.

According to Chinese medicine, your body is composed of energy, and, therefore, your body will respond positively or negatively to other energies within and also around you in the living world. In other words, everything within you and around you is all inter-connected through energy.

Energy healing began in China more than 5,000 years ago. At that time, some soldiers who received minor wounds inflicted on their bodies soon discovered that their physical pains and ailments had miraculously disappeared, and that led to the discovery of energy healing. The ancient Chinese physicians began to believe that there was an energy system in the human body, within which there was energy communication between different cells and organs. For centuries, the Chinese have believed that "qi" (the internal life energy) is responsible for transmitting energy information within the body. Accordingly, the smooth flow or stagnation of "qi" accounts for health or sickness.

Unlearning Diagnosis and Prognosis

In Latin, the word "doctor" means a "teacher." The role of the doctor is to "teach," and the role of the patient is to "learn." In other words, you are *also* responsible for your own health and healing.

A doctor's misdiagnosis of an illness may have a devastating impact on the patient, while a delayed diagnosis may negatively impact the prognosis of a disease. A doctor's diagnosis error may lead to incorrect treatment, delayed treatment, or no treatment at all; as a result, a patient's condition can be made much worse, and may even die.

There are many medical malpractice lawsuits, especially in the United States. The truth of the matter is that we *all* make mistakes, including doctors and medical experts.

Relearning Diagnosis and Prognosis

Prevention is always better than cure. If there is no disease, where is the need for a cure or even a doctor?

Take the step of maintaining optimal health and wellness in the body, the mind, and the soul, irrespective of your current conditions of health.

Nobody knows your body better than yourself; you have been living with it for years, if not decades. It is more than just treating a disease: it is also using that disease as a tool for understanding yourself— or, more specifically, *why* you are sick in the first place. It may give you the knowledge and wisdom to live in balance and harmony, thereby instrumental in initiating your healing with or without your doctor.

Remember, you do not have to follow any specific program or even the advice of anyone, maybe even including that of your doctor.

An Illustration

You need not follow the advice of former **President Bill Clinton** with respect to his dramatic weight loss—simply because you are not Bill Clinton, and your body's constitution is not the same as that of his. Therefore, what is good for Bill Clinton may not necessarily be good for yourself. Nor do you have to impose any deliberate discipline on yourself. The reason is that any imposition may stimulate your inherent resistant nature. Discovering your own sensitivity to life is often more important than rigidity.

The TAO

According to the TAO, an empty mind paves the way to both unlearning and relearning. Emptiness is synonymous with *simplicity* and *receiving*—the former is living a simple lifestyle with humility to develop an empty mindset to let go of all your attachments; the latter is the readiness and the capability to self-intuit true knowledge and profound wisdom.

On your healing journey, you need your compass and your roadmap. The compass is your wisdom, while the roadmap is only your knowledge. Wisdom, which is invisible, intangible, and invaluable, is emptiness, which comes only from an empty mind:

> "The spokes and the hub are the visible parts of a wheel.
> Clay is the visible material of a pot, which is useful because it contains.
> Walls, doors, and windows are visible parts of a house.
>
> We always look for the visible and the tangible without.
> But what really matters is the invisible and the intangible within."
> (Lao Tzu, **Tao Te Ching**, Chapter 11)

According to the TAO, to attain knowledge, add things every day, but to attain wisdom, remove things every day:

> "Seeking the Creator,
> we give up something every day.
> The less we have,
> the less we need to strain and strive
> until we need to do nothing.
> Allowing things to come and go,
> following their natural laws,
> we gain everything.
> Straining and striving,
> we lose everything."
> (Lao Tzu, **Tao Te Ching**, Chapter 48)

The explanation is that "less is for more" and not "more is for more" according to the contemporary thinking:

> "Without going out the door, we know the world.
> Without looking out the window, we see the Creator.
> The more we look outside ourselves,
> the less we know about anything.
>
> Trusting the Creator, the ancient prophets
> knew without doing, understood without seeing.
> Trusting the Creator, we accomplish without striving."
> (Lao Tzu, ***Tao Te Ching***, Chapter 47)

On your healing journey, you just have to learn, unlearn, and relearn from anyone, anything, and any situation:

> "Everything that happens to us is beneficial.
> Everything that we experience is instructional.
> Everyone that we meet, good or bad, becomes our teacher or student.
>
> We learn from both the good and the bad.
> So, stop picking and choosing.
> Everything is a manifestation of the mysteries
> of creation."
> (Lao Tzu, ***Tao Te Ching***, Chapter 27)

You do not set any goal or have any objective in your learning, unlearning, and relearning. The explanation is that setting any goal or having any objective will make you judge and choose, and thereby instrumental in pre-conditioning your thinking mind with respect to your learning, unlearning, and relearning:

"The foolish all have goals.
The wise are humble and stubborn.
They alone trust the Creator,
and not the world He created."
(Lao Tzu, *Tao Te Ching*, Chapter 20)

"Accepting what is, we find perfection in the Creator,
as well as in everything created by Him.

What seemingly distorted is in fact truthful.
What seemingly lacking is in fact abundant.
What seemingly exhausted is in fact refreshing.

Possessing little, we become content.
Having too much, we lose the Creator.
Having no ego, we become humbled, and our actions are enlightened.
Having no desire for perfection, our actions are welcome by all.
Having no expectation of result, our actions are selfless and non-judgmental.
Having no goal, our actions are under-doing and never over-doing.

Accepting what is, and finding it to be perfect

is not easy.
But that is the Way to the Creator."
(Lao Tzu, ***Tao Te Ching***, Chapter 22)

The Step of Discovery and Recovery

On your healing journey, unlearning and relearning may change your perspectives of *how* you look at your life and your health. This transformation may bring about your self-awakening discovery of how and why you might have your *myasthenia gravis*, as well as your ultimate recovery from it .

Discovery of Natural Self-Healing

Hippocrates (460 - 370 B.C), the father of medicine, once said: "Our food should be our medicine. Our medicine should be our food." Take a step further: Let food be the "only" medicine. If you have developed a degenerative disease, start thinking of food as your medicine, in fact, the best medicine, if not the "only" medicine. Your body is designed to digest and utilize food to get its nutrients and energy. But only wholesome food can do just that—not even supplements, because all supplements are just what they are called.

If food is the "only" medicine for you, you will empower yourself with knowledge about food, and you will then pursue a proper diet with high quality, non-toxic, and nutritious food. That means, you will refrain from eating the commercially-prepared and chemically-loaded food obtainable at supermarkets.

When food becomes the "only" medicine, you will also learn to trust your body; that is, you will learn what your body is telling you, and how it responds to real and wholesome food.

When you do become sick, you should also learn how to use herbs as medicine. Herbs from different parts of plants have different therapeutic values that promote self-healing without the use of dangerous pharmaceutical drugs. As a matter of fact, many common herbs, such as cinnamon, garlic, and ginger, have been used as "food" medicine for thousands of years.

According to a Chinese saying, "You can never draw a line between foods and herbs. Herbs can cure many common ailments, such as constipation, cholesterol, high blood pressure, with little or no side effects. For example, use ginger's anti-inflammatory properties to fight arthritis pain and nausea; use hawthorn berries for cardiovascular health; use aloe juice to cure an upset stomach.

If food is your "only" medicine, you will make good use of it to improve your health and heal yourself of any disease, including *myasthenia gravis*.

Hippocrates had also said: "Healing is a matter of time, but it is also a matter of opportunity." Therefore, give your body that opportunity for natural self-healing by going drug-free, although it may take more time.

Your life is a journey through which you make many choices—some good ones and also some bad ones—that contribute to your health or illnesses. Life has a purpose with a unique destiny for each individual. Therefore, it is important that you know yourself, and self-healing is "knowing the self" as a part of your destiny. Sometimes and somewhere along your life journey, you may hit rock bottom and begin to despair. You may even ask the frequently-asked question: "Why *me*?" But that may also be the time of self-awakening for you. You may then begin to question *how* and *why* you have found yourself in that difficult and despondent situation. True self-awakening will make you take a different path—a detour from that journey you have been prodding along. Taking a different path creates the energy for self-healing.

Your self-awakening can be physical, such as a change of diet or taking up an exercise regimen. Your self-wakening can be emotional or spiritual, such as self-awakening to the power of love and compassion. For example, through the self-healing power of meditation, you may be awakened to a new awareness of reality, a new consciousness of who you really are and what your priorities in life are. Self-awakening may give you the desire and intention to heal, precipitating in changes that will ultimately heal not just the body but also the mind. Your very desire to heal is the healing energy for the body and the mind.

If you know yourself well, you will empower your

mind with knowledge to heal yourself, and that empowerment generates more healing energy. If you know yourself more, you will make more right choices, than wrong ones, regarding your health. In making those right choices, you are well on the path to your own self-healing.

Unfortunately, many of us place the responsibility of healing on our doctors. We readily relinquish our own responsibility to know ourselves to bring about our own self-healing. As a result, we remain sick and unhealed. **Dr. Felix Marti-Ibanez**, M.D., hit the nail on the head when he wrote: "Only by knowing the healthy man can we cure him. . . . . To be a doctor, then, means much more than to dispense pills or to patch up torn flesh and shattered mind." What Dr. Marti-Ibanez meant was that you need to know yourself in order to be healed, because nobody knows your health better than yourself. Only you yourself can create that healing energy.

The bottom line: self-healing begins with knowing yourself through self-awakening to generate internal healing energy

Recovery of Natural Health

Myasthenia gravis is a disease or disorder caused by the malfunctioning of the immune system. It is partially a result of the accumulated toxins in the body, impairing and weakening the entire immune system.

It is an indisputable fact that pharmaceutical drugs are toxic chemicals. Although they may be effective in temporarily removing some of the undesirable symptoms of a disease, they also have long-term adverse side effects. Therefore, carefully consider the trade-off. The ultimate goal is always to eliminate the use of *all* pharmaceutical drugs.

Detoxification

Detoxification is internal cleansing, which involves *dislodging* your body toxins and waste products from within, as well as between cells and joints, and then *transporting* these wastes from your body for their ultimate removal.

Sources of toxins

All these years, knowingly or unknowingly, you may have poisoned your own body with toxins coming from many different sources: industrial wastes; pesticides and herbicides from agricultural products; exhaust fumes from factories and automobiles; food contamination; toxic pharmaceutical drugs; polluted waters; irradiation from excess use of cell phones, microwave ovens, power plants, radio and satellite transmissions; chemicals in food processing; toxic emotions and negative thoughts. Your body may have ingested all these toxins through *absorption*, *consumption*, *inhalation*, and *radiation*, creating health hazards to your immune system. All these toxins have accumulated and remained in your body.

Heavy metals, such as aluminum, cadmium, lead, and mercury, can also cause damages to your immune system. Minerals, which make up approximately four percent of your total body weight, are essential for your immune system and energy production. However, heavy metals can also damage your DNA, adversely change the neurons in your brain, elevate your cholesterol level and blood pressure, as well as deplete your bones of calcium and other minerals. They all play a pivotal role in damaging your immune system, leading to the development of your *myasthenia gravis*.

Common symptoms of a toxic body

The toxins in your body may manifest themselves physically, mentally, and spiritually in the form of bad breath, chronic constipation, chronic fatigue, frequent gas and bloating, hemorrhoids, irritability, mental and spiritual lethargy, overweight, mental depression, and recurrent headaches or migraines.

These symptoms should not be taken lightly: they often indicate imbalance in the body that may affect your immune system, and thus further aggravating your *myasthenia gravis* symptoms.

Ways of detoxification

There are different ways by which your body can get rid of its toxins:

- Fasting to detoxify

    Fasting is internal cleansing and health rejuvenation—one of the most effective and efficient ways to detoxify your body of its toxins. Fasting is to recovery, as sleep is to recuperation.

    Fasting is *voluntary* abstinence from food and drink, except water, for an extended period. Fasting is the *best* way to detoxify your body.

    The benefits of fasting

    Fasting has many health benefits, especially for the immune system.

    Fasting activates your immune system to protect you from diseases, especially the development of an autoimmune disease.

    Fasting accelerates the *self-healing* process of your body because it temporarily stops the continuing work of your digestive system, and therefore instrumental in reserving that energy for your internal self-healing process. By conserving the energy otherwise used in digesting food, fasting provides you with *more*, and not less, energy, contrary to the myth that fasting makes your body weak. Remember, eating and digesting food expends your energy too.

Fasting relieves the burden of not only your digestive tract, but also your liver and kidneys, which have to work extra hard to remove additives and toxins accumulated in your body through improper eating. Fasting removes the underlying cause of any *chronic disease* you may have by removing the toxins, not just the symptoms as in the case of medications.

Fasting may alleviate your *body pain* and rid your body of any drug dependence. Fasting facilitates you, if you are a smoker, to quit smoking during a fast. Nicotine damages the immune system.

The process of fasting

Eat more vegetables and fruits prior to a fast. Reduce the consumption of meat, and refrain from eating any meat the day before a fast.

On the *first* day, you may feel pangs of hunger, with a white coating on your tongue. This is just a natural response of the body to the cessation of eating. On the first day, you may even experience physical weakness, hunger, and food craving. The first day of a fast is most challenging and difficult to endure.

On the *second* day, you may begin to feel gradual dissipation of hunger, with more white coating on your tongue. The discomfort is less severe than the first day of your fast

On the *third* day you may or may not feel *complete* disappearance of hunger and the clearance of coating on your tongue.

The first three days of a fast are most difficult and challenging. However, once that period is overcome, you are well on the way to rejuvenation of your entire body. After the first three days, you do NOT feel any hunger, and that is the truth about fasting. The only hurdle you need to overcome is the first three days of your fast. Remember, **Jesus**, too, fasted for forty days.

What to do during a fast

Drinking plenty of water is required since your body may easily become dehydrated due to the discharge of your body fluids.

Continue your normal daily routine activities, but avoid all strenuous activities, especially those outdoor ones. Exercise as normal.

Bathe more frequently. Brush your body to stimulate your skin to rid toxins from your body.

Stop taking your daily vitamin supplements while you are fasting.

Consult your doctor to see if you may stop some of the medications you are currently taking.

Stop smoking if you are a smoker. Now is as good a time as any to quit smoking for good.

How to break a fast

Break a fast with fruits and vegetables juice. Eating an apple is ideal for breaking a fast.

Continue to drink plenty of water after a fast.

Gradually increase your intake of solid food. Eat slowly and chew thoroughly. Overeating too soon may cause abdominal pain and even vomiting.

Avoid taking salt and pepper immediately after a fast, lest they damage your stomach lining.

Remember, the longer the fast, the less you should eat at the *first* meal.

Duration of a fast

A *clear* tongue and *clean* breath are good indications that the cleansing is more or less complete.

The length of a fast depends very much on each individual. The following is just a general guideline for you to follow:

A one-day fast as often as required, preferably weekly, for good health maintenance

A three-to-four-day fast several times a year for general health and well-being

A two-week fast every year or so for complete internal cleansing

A three-week fast (or even longer) for curing a specific disease, under the supervision of a physician.

It is suggested that you begin with a short fast first, and then proceed to a longer fast for complete internal cleansing of your whole body.

- Breathing to detoxify

Breathing is the only body function that you can always perform both consciously and unconsciously.

The way you breathe is connected to your body and mind. For example, when you are anxious or angry, your breathing becomes quick and shallow—that reduces your body's natural capability to detoxify.

You can *consciously* change your breathing patterns to relax your body and mind to enhance detoxification, for example practicing *diaphragm breathing* (see **page 54**). By holding in your abdominal muscles while pushing out your lower rib cage to expand your diaphragm in your inhalation, you not only acquire *complete breath* (that is, inhaling more oxygen) but also achieve internal cleansing by pumping more lymphatic fluid throughout the body and circulatory systems.

- Skin brushing to detoxify

   Skin brushing, an external way to detoxify the body, is an effective time-honored method to increase blood and lymphatic circulation to remove dead skin cells, and rid your body of toxins, especially through its pores.

   Brush your entire body daily with a natural-bristle dry-skin brush. Be persistent, and the initial discomfort will dissipate after a while when your body has become accustomed to the abrasive effects of brushing.

- Foot patches to detoxify

   The use of foot patches is an easy and unobtrusive way to assist your body in the removal of a myriad of pollutants that invade your body on a daily basis, as well as the health-repressive toxins that prevent your body from achieving the true wellness you should really be experiencing.

According to the Chinese medical knowledge, the human body has over 360 acupuncture points, with more than 60 of them found on the *soles* of the feet alone. Your feet, also known as the "second heart", contain the reflective zones of your internal organs, where your body toxins accumulate and dissipate.

For centuries, many Chinese medical studies have held the view that due to gravity, toxins tend to go downward in your body during the whole day, accumulating from the tips of the toes to the ankles.

Accordingly, when applied to the soles of your feet *overnight*, these foot patches not only warm up to open pores of the skin but also stimulate the reflex zones on your soles to draw out and absorb accumulated wastes from the blood and lymph systems in your body under osmotic pressure.

When lying horizontally, your body fluids collect in your head and feet. There is an acupuncture point on each of the sole of your feet, known as "gushing water spring", through which excess toxins and moisture from your body will be excreted into the foot patches. By applying foot patches on your feet while sleeping, you may be able to extract toxins from your body through the process of osmosis in the form of moisture onto your soles, and then into the foot patches.

Foot patches are obtainable on the Internet or in Chinese drug stores. Get them to remove toxins from your body.

- Hydrotherapy to detoxify

    Water is an invaluable nutrient to every living thing on earth. Every cell of your body requires water to carry nutrients and energy to it, as well as to transport toxins and waste products from it.

    Always drink enough water. Drink a cup of water as soon as you get up in the morning, not your tea or coffee as your first drink.

    According to a survey, only 30 percent of Americans drink at least eight eight-ounce glasses of water a day. Make sure you drink *enough* water, which is more than eight eight-ounce glasses a day. One of the main reasons why people do not drink enough water is that they do not enjoy the taste of plain water; another reason is that they do not have the time, especially if they do not feel thirsty (when they *feel* thirsty, they are already dehydrated without knowing it).

According to the Human Nutrition Center at Rockefeller University, water is the best choice for proper hydration.

Drink water on schedule, such as every two hours or so, even if you do not feel thirsty.

Avoid all pasteurized and processed fruit juices, carbonated beverages with artificial sweeteners and additives, and all dehydrating beverages, such as coffee, tea, sodas, beer, wine and other alcoholic drinks.

The bottom line: drink more water to flush out toxins for internal cleansing.

Unclean water is damaging to health. Always drink only pure water in order to reduce the load on your liver.

When you drink commercial water with additives, carbonation, artificial flavorings, and sweeteners, your liver must also work *overtime* to filter them before the water can be absorbed by your body to carry out its proper functions, one of which is to flush out the toxins and wastes from your body system.

The circulating system of blood and lymphatic fluids is vital to all your organs, tissues, and cells in that it enables the removal of waste products from your body.

Hydrotherapy involves alternating application of hot and cold water aimed at increasing your blood flow to different tissues of your body. Take a very hot shower immediately followed by a very cold one, and repeat the process two or three times a day. After the hydrotherapy, snuggle into your bed, staying warm for at least half an hour or so. With hydrotherapy, you will feel completely refreshed and rejuvenated.

Hydrotherapy provides detoxification benefits to your entire circulating system:

The alternating hot and cold water opens up pores in your skin for more effective elimination.

Blood flow increases circulation to your intestines in the abdomen (an empty stomach yielding the best result), thereby promoting digestion.

The filtering organs of your chest and abdomen are relaxed through the induced circulation.

The nerves along your spinal cord also become stimulated and relaxed.

- Exercise to detoxify

    Exercise not only stimulates blood circulation and the movement of lymphatic fluids, but also promotes the reduction of fat reserves, thereby instrumental in facilitating the removal of toxins stored in your body.

    Low-impact aerobic exercise, such as jumping rope or on a bouncer, can significantly improve your body's circulation to enhance detoxification.

    Understandably, your weak muscles may make it difficult for you to exercise. Do simple Yoga, Tai-Chi, or Qi-Gong exercises not only to promote flexibility of muscles but also to increase muscular strength.

- Foods to detoxify

    Use foods for regular body detoxification, further rejuvenation, and daily maintenance. Some of the top detox foods to help your immune system are as follows:

    Apple

    An apple a day keeps the doctor away. There is much truth in that: apple is a powerful antioxidant and toxin remover due to its vitamin C and its fiber and pectin. Eat an apple every day to keep your immune system healthy and strong.

Alfalfa sprouts

Alfalfa sprouts are excellent "health food." Recent research shows that in addition to being a superb source of nutrients, they also have important *cleansing* ability due to their concentrated amounts of phytochemical (plant compounds).

You can grow your own alfalfa sprouts at your home. Just buy some organic alfalfa seeds, put them in a jar, wash and rinse them two or three times a day, and you will have your fresh sprouts in a few days. Sprout some alfalfa seeds at home for your daily salad or soup.

Fresh alfalfa sprouts are also obtainable at some supermarkets.

Artichoke

Artichoke increases your bile production to facilitate your bowel movement. Steam artichoke and serve with a little melted butter.

Avocado

Avocado is rich in glutathione antioxidant, which is effective in removing toxins due to too much alcohol consumption. Eat an avocado for breakfast; it is filling and saves you time.

Beets

Beets help you detoxify your *liver* and *blood* while providing important support nutrients to your body. By providing nutrients critical to liver function and healthy kidneys, beets break down toxins before they accumulate in your liver. In addition, the vitamins and other nutrients contained in beets enable proper fat absorption, transportation, and metabolism. Include fresh beets in your vegetable juice or salad.

Burdock

Burdock, a carrot-like root grown in China, Europe, and the United States, has a sweet taste and a sticky texture. It is a good source of minerals and essential oils. As such, burdock serves as a staple vegetable in Japan.

Burdock, with its potent anti-bacterial and anti-fungal properties, is a popular folk medicine around the world. As a main source for a variety of herbal preparations, it serves also as a diuretic and, more recently, as a tea to fight cancer (*Essiac* tea in the treatment of cancer and a number of other maladies).

Burdock is a potent "blood purifier" which clears toxins from your bloodstream by enhancing the function of many organs of elimination, including your liver, kidneys and bowels. For example, it induces sweating as an aid in neutralizing and eliminating toxins, thereby instrumental in helping your kidneys filter uric acid from your bloodstream.

Put fresh burdock in your soup, or make a drink of burdock by simmering it in boiling water for 10 minutes (you can repeat the process until its taste is gone). Daily consumption of burdock is recommended for your daily internal cleansing.

Green barley

The young barley leaf is a green cereal grass that contains the greatest and most balanced concentration of nutrients found in nature: enzymes, minerals, many vitamins, including vitamin C, vitamin A, and B vitamins, amino acids, essential fatty acids, carotenoids, bioflavonoids and chlorophyll. The chlorophyll in green barley has the ability to break down carbon dioxide and release oxygen, thereby enabling the destruction of anaerobic bacteria. Green barley, in addition to its natural form, is available in capsules or powder.

Cruciferous vegetables

Brussels sprouts, cabbage, cauliflower, and spinach are all effective in enhancing your liver in its production of enzymes for your digestion and elimination. Eat them as much and as often as you can, either cooked or raw.

Garlic

Garlic contains allicin, which is a potent purifier of mercury and other toxic chemicals found in most food additives. In addition, garlic alkalizes the body, making it more efficient in resisting disease. Put crushed garlic in all your cooking. If you wish to remove the odor from the unpleasant breath due to garlic, chew some fresh parsley for a fresher breath.

Kiwi fruit

Like avocado, kiwi fruit is loaded with glutathione. In addition, it is rich in vitamin C. It is also a powerful antioxidant to protect your immune system.

Seaweed

Seaweed contains high doses of minerals, such as calcium, iodine, iron, and magnesium, according to a research at McGill University in Canada. Seaweed is an inexpensive sea vegetable. Use seaweed in your daily soup.

Watercress

Watercress increases detox enzymes in your body for internal cleansing. Watercress is especially effective in removing carcinogens from smokers, according to a United Kingdom research study. Steam or put watercress in your soup.

- Herbs to detoxify

    Your body is a self-cleaning mechanism, which utilizes your liver, kidneys, urine, feces, breath, and sweat to detoxify your toxins.

    Herbs can provide you with safe, natural, and time-tested ways to improve the natural functions of your body through their natural cleansing processes.

    Some of the most common herbs for detoxification include: black walnut, cascara sagrada, cayenne, dandelion, echinacea, fennel seed, Indian rhubarb root, licorice root, milk thistle, psyllium husk, red clover, slipper elm inner bark, and yarrow. All these herbs can be obtained on the Internet.

Holistic detoxification

For detoxification to be effective, a holistic approach is required. The body, the mind, and the spirit of an individual are all inter-connected.

For this reason, holistic detoxification is the only way to optimum self-cleansing for a healthy immune system.

The spirit also plays an important role. Fasting, for example, is more than a matter of willpower: it involves a deepening of faith and the capability to let go. Fasting is a spiritual act of the mind to detoxify the body. The spirit affects how you react to anger, anxiety, frustration, and other everyday negative emotions that may adversely increase the toxicity in your body because your toxic thoughts are stored in your subconscious mind, which in turn controls your conscious mind. You are what you think: you become your toxic thoughts. Therefore, the role of the spirit in holistic detoxification cannot be overstressed.

The TAO

According to the TAO, your discovery in life is your effortless search for learning and teaching from unexpected people in unexpected places; your recovery is your subjective perception of all the connections of life with your own spontaneous flow with them. Embracing everything and everyone with no judgment and no preference is the way to the discovery and the recovery of your health.

"The Way is paradoxical.
Like water, soft and yielding,
yet it overcomes the hard and the rigid.
Stiffness and stubbornness cause much suffering.

We all intuitively know
that flexibility and tenderness
are the Way to go.
Yet our conditioned mind
tells us to go the other way.

We accept all that is simple and humble.
We embrace the good fortune and the misfortune.
Thus, we become masters of every situation.
We overcome the painful and the difficult in our lives.
That is why the Way seems paradoxical."
(Lao Tzu, ***Tao Te Ching***, Chapter 78)

The recovery journey is never smooth and straightforward; it is always long and winding, with many detours and even setbacks. Healing is invisible, inaudible, and intangible:

"Look, it is invisible.
Listen, it is inaudible.
Grab, it is intangible.

These three characteristics are indefinable:
Therefore, they are joined as one, just like the Creator—invisible, inaudible, and intangible.

As one, it is unbroken thread with neither a beginning nor an end.
It returns to nothingness: invisible, inaudible, and intangible.
It is the indefinable, the intangible, and the unimaginable.
Stand before it, and there is no beginning.
Follow it, and there is no end.
Only by its grace can we discover how things have been and will be.
This is the essence of the Creator: invisible, inaudible, and intangible."
(Lao Tzu, **Tao Te Ching**, Chapter 14)

"Only with His grace do we find renewal and rebirth along the Way."
(Lao Tzu, **Tao Te Ching**, Chapter 5)

Recovery has much to do with moderation, meaning prevention, which is always better than cure:

"With the golden mean, there is moderation.
With moderation, our limits are unknown.
With unknown limits, our potentials are infinite.
With infinite potentials, our power is everlasting.
With the golden mean, we accommodate ourselves to
the ever-changing world around us.
We simplify the complicated with gentle ease,
like a mother caring for her child.

Deep rooted in the presence of the golden mean,
we follow the Way, and never lose our way."
(Lao Tzu, **Tao Te Ching**, Chapter 59)

With the discovery of your own health conditions, your recovery is easy to find and follow:

"The Way is easy to find and follow:
empty the mind of conditioned thinking
of seeing things and doing things.

The Way comes from the source of all.
Its power cherishes and nourishes all.
Knowing the source, we know ourselves.

Finding the Way,
we know the nature of things;
we see the comings and goings of things.

Following the Way,
we discover the treasures within;
we simplify the trappings without.
So, we continue the Way with inner joy."
(Lao Tzu, **Tao Te Ching**, Chapter 70)

The Step of Maintenance and Sustenance

Now that your body has been cleansed inside out, it is important to maintain it in optimum conditions also inside out.

To do just that, you have to listen to your body,

before and after you eat. That is, physiologically, what you eat immediately affects your body's cell reparation, while, psychologically and spiritually, your food ingredients may also affect how you feel and think.

Given the optimum environment, your body cells can replicate themselves throughout your lifespan because they are most resilient and rejuvenating.

If you have reduced or stopped your medications, and you have also been detoxifying your body, now is the time to use foods as your medicine for maintenance and sustenance to further promote your ongoing self-healing process.

Acid-Alkaline Balance

Your body cells need an optimum environment for replication and rejuvenation. They need a balanced acid-and-alkaline environment.

Acid and alkaline are substances that have opposing qualities. Your body functions at its best when the pH is optimum, which is slightly alkaline. The pH of your blood, tissues, and body fluids directly affects the state of your cellular health, and hence your immune system, which plays a pivotal role in the continual healing of your *myasthenia gravis*.

The pH scale ranges between one and fourteen. *Seven* is considered neutral. Anything *below* seven is considered *acidic*, while anything *above* seven is considered *alkaline*. Deviations above or below a 7.30 and 7.40 pH range can signal potentially serious and dangerous symptoms, forewarning you of a disease in process.

When your body is too acidic, the tissues of your cells are forced to relinquish their alkaline reserves, depleting them of alkaline minerals, which are the components of the tissues themselves.

The acute shortage of alkaline minerals will lead to disease and the malfunctioning of the immune system, causing an autoimmune disease, including *myasthenia gravis*.

Acidification

Acidification may come from the following:

- Excess intake of foods containing great amounts of acid

- Insufficient elimination of acid by the body through the kidneys (urination) and the skin (sweating).

Not too much acid can actually stay in the bloodstream, and, accordingly, any excess is then directed to other body organs and tissues, where it can accumulate. Too much acidification makes your body become sick:

- Acid corrosion

    The corrosive nature of acid irritates your body organs, causing inflammation (which is often a source of body pain), pain, and hardening of tissues.

    Acidic sweat may cause skin allergy, especially in areas where sweat seems to accumulate, such as the armpits.

    Acidic urine may also cause infection and inflammation in the urinary tract, resulting in bladder problems.

    Acidification not only causes lesions of the mucous membranes (e.g. your respiratory system), making them more vulnerable to infections, but also impairs the immune system.

- Decreased enzyme activity

    Acidification decreases the activity of enzymes in the body, which are responsible for proper digestion of foods and assimilation of nutrients.

- Loss of minerals

    Loss of minerals may result in: bone loss (osteoporosis); brittle bones (hip fracture); joint inflammation (arthritis); hair loss (baldness); split fingernails; dry skin, and wrinkles.

Sources of Acidification

Contemporary lifestyle is the main cause of excess acidification in body cells, which may ultimately lead to diseases.

- Diet

    Diet is the main contributor to excess acidification in the body. The main sources of acid from foods are: cereals (good for the food industry, not for the health); sugars (bad for the body's metabolism); animal proteins (difficult for digestion and assimilation by the body).

    The main sources of acidification from drinks are: alcohol, coffee, sodas, sugary drinks (often disguised as health drinks), and tea.

- Tobacco

    Tobacco smoke causes acidification in the respiratory system. Quit smoking now, if you are still a smoker!

- Exercise

    Too much exercise (more may not be better), or the lack of it, may lead to acidification.

- Stress

    Stress in everyday life and living may cause physiological disturbances, often resulting in acidification of your body system.

Diseases caused by acidification

Diseases caused by too much acidification are related to the following:

- The immune system

- The skin—allergies and rashes

- The respiratory system—bronchitis, colds, flu, laryngitis

- The nervous system—chronic fatigue, mental depression (due to deficiency in alkaline minerals, including calcium, magnesium, and potassium)

- The urinary system (due to lesions in mucous membranes of the urinary tract).

Acidification is often the inability of the body to metabolize a particular nutrient, such as sugar and animal protein. The wisdom is to avoid sugar totally and to reduce the intake of animal protein, both of which are the main culprits of excess acidification in the body.

Foods rich in weak acids, such as fruits, vinegar, and yogurt, are normally quite easy to oxidize, contributing to a large number of alkaline elements in the body. However, if you experience poor oxidation in these foods, your metabolism debility may then make you more prone to acidification. There are certainly no hard-and-fast rules governing how these weak-acid foods may become either acidic or alkaline for different individuals.

The bottom line: get rid of your sugar addiction.

Symptoms of excess acidification

Too much acid in your body may result in some of the following symptoms: acid regurgitation; acidic sweat or dry skin; brittle and fungal nails; conjunctivitis; cracks at the corners of the lips; diarrhea; frequent headaches; insomnia; irritability; leg crams and spasms; lack of energy; lower body temperature; pimples; runny nose; and weight loss.

Measuring and changing acid-alkaline levels

Measure the acid-alkaline levels in you body by performing a simple urine test with litmus paper (obtainable at pharmacies).

Reduce or eliminate acidification in your body by the following:

- Change your lifestyle: make it *less* stressful.

- Adjust your diet for more alkaline foods and drinks.

- Consume medicinal plants to promote the flow of your urine (diuretics) and to increase the production of sweat.

- Take daily alkaline mineral supplements to facilitate internal cleansing.

- Go on a regular water or juice fast to enhance the elimination of toxins lodged in the deep tissues of your body.

- Exercise moderately to prevent acidification.

Foods to balance acid-alkaline levels

Your diet is the primary source that determines your acid-alkaline levels in your body.

Always choose the right foods for better body chemistry for better immunity health.

Acidifying foods

Acidifying foods are characterized by their high protein content, and/or fats, including the following: meat, poultry, fish and seafood; eggs; cheese; vegetable oils; whole grains; beans, such as broad bean, chickpeas, peanuts, soybeans, and white beans; bread, pasta, and cereals; sweets and sugars, including brown sugar and honey; sugary drinks and sodas; alcohol, coffee, and tea.

Your digestion of protein produces amino acids (containing acid minerals, such as phosphorus and sulfur) during digestion, and uric acids during acidic degradation.

You utilize fat in the form of fatty acids, and your digestion of saturated fat is often incomplete, resulting in toxic acid substances that contribute to acidification.

Your digestion of glucose may be adversely affected by inadequate or poor metabolism, turning originally alkaline elements into acidic ones.

Your consumption of too much sugar strains your body metabolism in converting it into energy, and thus creating more acid in the process.

The bottom line: consume *less* acidifying foods.

Acid foods may be alkalizing if your body's metabolism is efficient. In other words, if your body can easily metabolize and oxidize them, these foods can be transformed into alkaline elements, making your body more alkaline, instead of more acidic.

Acid foods contain a good deal of acid, and are acidic in taste, including the following: blueberries, raspberries, and strawberries; oranges, grapefruit, lemons, Mandarin oranges, and tangerines; sweet fruits, such as watermelon; unripe fruits; acid vegetables, such as rhubarb, tomato, and watercress; honey; vinegar; and yogurt.

Always eat the fruit, instead of drinking its juice. The reason is that alkaline minerals are present in the pulp; the juice without the pulp is only more acidic. Cooking fruits does not remove their acidity.

Alkalizing foods, on the other hand, contain little or no acid substances, and they do not produce acids when metabolized by your body. Alkalizing foods include the following: green vegetables; colored vegetables (except tomato); chestnut; potato; avocado; black olives; bananas; dried fruits; almonds and Brazil nuts; milk; alkaline mineral waters; and cold-pressed oils.

Potato, especially its juice, is good for stomach acidity and ulcers. It is often an ideal alternative to acidifying cereal grains.

Dried fruits are alkalizing because much of the acid is removed through the drying process. Eat more dried fruits.

Alkalizing medicinal plants

Black currant fruits are a good source of vitamin C and other vitamins and minerals, including an omega-6 fatty acid to increase blood flow, to decrease blood clotting, and to reduce inflammation (often a source of many types of body pain).

Black currant seed oil is especially good for rheumatoid arthritis (an autoimmune disease), due to its anti-inflammatory properties in decreasing the morning stiffness in the joints.

According to the *British Journal of Rheumatology*, black currant oil is effective because of a reduction in the secretion of the inflammatory cytokines (a source of inflammation).

Black currant seed oil is also beneficial to cardiovascular disease due to the presence of its omega-6 fatty acids.

Black currant seed oil helps reduce the severity of menstrual cramps due to the inflammatory omega-6 fatty acids.

According to the Skin Study Center in Philadelphia, black currant seed oil helps with dry skin disorders. The gamma-linoleic acid (GLA) in black currant protects against water loss that contributes to itching and other symptoms associated with dry skin.

Burdock is a plant native to Asia and Europe, which has become available to all parts of the world. Ancient Chinese and Indian herbalists always used burdock to treat respiratory infections, abscesses, and joint pain. The root of burdock is one of the primary sources of most herbal preparations. Eat burdock every day to have a healthy immune system to eliminate many of the symptoms of your *myasthenia gravis*

Cranberry has been in use since the Iron Age, but the Romans were the first to recognize its medicinal values. Cranberry, which is high in vitamin C and antioxidants, contains anti-asthmatic compounds.

Scientific studies have shown cranberry to be effective in helping to prevent or eliminate urinary tract infections. This berry is useful in fighting yeast infections, as well as kidney stones and chronic kidney inflammation.

According to a study reported at the 2006 International Association for Dental Research's 84th General Session & Exhibition in Brisbane, Australia, the antioxidant properties of cranberry help fight dental plaque.

Alkalizing energy boosters

Spirulina is a green alga, rich in chlorophyll, containing the highest protein and beta-carotene levels of all green super foods. It is the highest known vegetable source of B-12, minerals, trace elements, cell salts, amino acids, DNA and RNA, and enzymes.

Spirulina helps with digestion, elimination, detoxification, internal cleansing, tissue repair, skin problems, healing and prevention of degenerative diseases. It also promotes longevity. Spirulina is effective in any weight-control diet because its high nutritional value helps satisfying the hidden hunger or deficiencies.

Blackstrap molasses is an excellent source of iron and calcium, copper, magnesium, manganese, and potassium. It can even reverse grey hair due to its copper content.

Make a healthy drink with a tablespoon of organic blackstrap molasses (mixed in some hot water first) and ¾ cup of soymilk. Add ice.

Cod liver oil, which comes from fatty fish, such as salmon and sardines, is rich in vitamin A and vitamin D, and essential omega 3 oils. It enhances the absorption of calcium and maintains a constant level of blood calcium. Cod liver oil also improves brain functions and the nervous system.

In 2005, researchers at the University of California reported that vitamin D might lower the risk of developing different types of cancers, cutting in half the chances of getting breast, ovarian, or colon cancer.

Alkaline supplements

Alkaline supplements should contain calcium (Ca), sodium (Na), silica and copper, and other minerals to help de-acidification of your body. More importantly, they should contain every mineral in similar proportion to that found in the human body.

Remember, your body functions synergistically: that is, the whole is greater than the sum of its parts. Every mineral has a crucial role to play in the human anatomy.

Supplement your diet with coral calcium to keep all mineral levels up, as well as in their proper balance.

Avoid Food Allergies

Besides using foods to boost and enhance immune system health, it is also important to avoid food allergies.

Research has indicated that many autoimmune disease patients also have food allergies. This research finding of higher rates of allergies in general has led some experts to believe that food allergies may also be the triggering of some autoimmune diseases. Many nutritionists also concur that an anti-inflammatory diet not only may avoid getting another autoimmune disease, but also can alleviate some of the symptoms of an already-existing autoimmune disease.

Avoid Gastrointestinal Tract Infection

Make sure your gastrointestinal tract is thriving. Although your autoimmune disease, such as *myasthenia gravis*, is not directly connected to your stomach, your digestive health is inextricably linked to the source of your autoimmunity. In an unhealthy intestine, the lining may become impaired, and thus allowing larger molecules, such as bacteria and any undigested food particle, to slip through into the bloodstream. This may trigger an immune reaction.

Therefore, it is also important to cleanse your gastrointestinal tract through diet to prevent antigens from getting into your body system that may further increase the production of antibodies to go after the added antigens, and thus worsening your immune-driven disease symptoms.

Basics of Eating for a Healthy Immune System

There are basics of healthy eating; with a little discipline, they are simple to follow, and may go a long way to improving your immune system.

Eating to live, not living to eat

You become your foods, and your foods become you, because you are what you eat. What you eat and drink becomes your body chemistry.

Eating less, not more

Follow the "three-quarters" rule of eating: stop eating when you are three-quarters full. Never overeat.

Eating frequently, not three times a day

You need not follow the habit of eating three times a

day. Eat only when you are hungry, not because it is time to eat. Eating smaller meals more frequently is less taxing on your digestive and metabolic systems.

Eating living foods, not dead foods

Eat only living foods: fresh, whole, and, preferably, organic foods.

Do not eat processed foods (supermarket foods), which are loaded with colorings, preservatives, and taste enhancers.

Do not eat empty-calorie foods, such as white flour and white sugar: foods are supposed to give you energy and nutrients, not just empty calories.

Stop eating foods that damage your thyroid, which is critical to your immune health. Avoid foods that contain goitrogens, which are substances occurring naturally in certain foods that may cause your thyroid gland (goiter) to enlarge. Goitrogens are naturally found in soy, millet, coffee, and cruciferous vegetables, such as broccoli, cauliflower, cabbage, and kale (do not over-consume them; steam them instead of eating them raw). To enhance your thyroid health, take iodized salt (but not too much) and coconut oil. Also, drink plenty of water.

Eating sea salt, not table salt

Eat sea salt, which is loaded with minerals. Avoid

table salt. Research has shown that increased salt intake proportionately increases cancer risk in the bladder, esophagus, and stomach.

Eating no refined sugar

Get your sugar from fruits and vegetables. Stay away from refined sugar.

Artificial sugars, such as aspartame, saccharin, or sucralose, are more dangerous than refined sugar, because they are loaded with chemicals that impair the immune system. Stop your sugar craving and addiction!

Eating raw occasionally

For optimum digestion, your body needs enzymes, which are destroyed by heat in cooking. You need not be a vegetarian to go on raw, but vegetarians generally have a better and healthier immune system. An occasional raw diet increases enzyme activities for better digestion and assimilation to enhance your immune system.

Chewing thoroughly

Chew your food thoroughly—at least 20 times before swallowing. The health benefits of thorough chewing are:

- Activating enzymes for better digestion

- Facilitating the absorption of vitamins and nutrients

- Feeling fuller, therefore eating less (better weight control)

- Reducing the production of stomach acid (cause of heartburn).

Smart cooking

Steaming is the best way to cook. Steam your food to preserve its nutrients. The next best cooking method is stir-fry. Boiling destroys half of the vitamins in vegetables. Deep-frying not only yields fatty foods but also produces trans fat (the worst kind of fat).

Foods for the Immune System

Chlorella

Chlorella is a green single-cell alga cultivated in fresh water ponds. It is one of the best foods for the immune system.

- It has high concentration of chlorophyll.

- It has high source of protein.

- It is the perfect anti-aging food (more than 20 vitamins and minerals, with the essential eight amino acids) for overall health.

- It detoxifies by removing toxins and metals from the body.

Wheat grass

Wheat grass is another life-giving food for the immune system.

- It is rich in chlorophyll to provide oxygen for the brain and body tissues.

- It is loaded with enzymes for optimum digestion.

- It absorbs as many as 92 of the known 102 anti-aging minerals from the soil (if grown in organic soil) to boost your immune system.

Wheat grass juice is particularly a superior detoxification agent compared to carrot juice. It enhances digestion, relieves sore throat, keeps the bowels open, reduces blood pressure, and improves the cholesterol levels. Make your own wheat grass juice, or obtain it from a health food store.

Foods to Boost the Immune System

Apples

An apple a day keeps the doctor away. Eat two to three apples a day to keep you healthier for longer.

The pectin in apples may do wonders to your health by decreasing your cholesterol levels, facilitating your bowel movements to keep you internally clean, improving lung functions (according to one study, better lung function with eating at least five apples a week), and preventing colon cancer.

Brown Rice

Brown rice is one of the few pain-safe foods (foods that do not trigger body pain). It is one of the best staple foods for lowering high blood sugar (excellent for diabetics), and anti-aging (over 70 oxidants) with vitamin E, glutathione peroxidase, and coenzyme Q-10.

Do not eat white rice, which is stripped of some of its major nutrients.

Garlic

Eat fresh garlic every day. To overcome its pungency, chew some fresh parsley (rich in vitamin C). The allicin in garlic has the following medicinal properties: combating cancer, lowering cholesterol, preventing atherosclerosis and coronary blockage, reducing blood clot formation, regulating blood sugar, and stimulating the pituitary to produce hormones.

Sea Vegetables

Sea vegetables have more concentrated nutrients

(e.g. calcium, iron, and protein) than land vegetables.

Sea vegetables have immense health benefits for the immune system by detoxifying heavy metals, dissolving cysts and tumors, shrinking goiters, and reducing water retention for weight loss.

Add sea vegetables to your salads and soups.

Sweet Potatoes and yams

Sweet potatoes and yams are rich in beta-carotene, fiber, protein, vitamin C, and DHEA, which is a precursor hormone (dehydroepiandrosterone).

Drinks to Heal the Immune System

Burdock and daikon drink

Burdock root has been used as both food and medicine in Asia and Europe for thousands of years. Recently, it has been used as a nourishing tonic for cancer, liver disease, and rheumatism. Burdock root is a staple diet of the Japanese, who are among the people with the longest lifespan in the world.

Fresh burdock root is available at many greengrocers, Asian supermarkets, and natural food stores in the United States.

Daikon is Japanese radish. Its phytochemicals have

well-recognized healing and anti-carcinogenic properties:

- It cleanses the blood (the kidneys).

- It promotes energy circulation.

- It increases the metabolic rate (a weight-loss remedy in Asia).

- It treats hangovers.

- It decongests the lungs, clears sore throat, colds, and edema.

The burdock and daikon drink can be taken any time, and as much as you like.

Ingredients

- One burdock root (about 24 inches long)

- One daikon with green tops

- One small carrot with green tops.

Preparation

- Cut all ingredients into small pieces.

- Place them in a pot with water double the volume of the ingredients.

- Bring to a boil.

- Pour out the content, and drink it.

- You can repeat the process one more time. This time, after bringing it to a boil, reduce heat, and simmer it for another 20 minutes. Let the ingredients steep in the hot water for another 20 minutes before drinking it.

Four greens drink

Bitter melon, a popular Asian vegetable, is well known for blood glucose control. It contains a substance similar to bovine insulin, which has been shown in experimental studies to achieve a positive sugar regulating effect by suppressing the neural response to sweet taste stimuli.

Celery is a good source of insoluble fiber as well as essential nutrients, including vitamin C, calcium, and potassium. In addition, it may reduce blood pressure, and block cancer cells.

Cucumber has been associated with healing properties in relation to diseases of the kidney, urinary bladder, liver, and pancreas. In addition, cucumber juice is an excellent skin tonic.

Green pepper is loaded with vitamin C (a potent antioxidant) and beta-carotene (to prevent cataracts).

Make the nutritious four greens drink by juicing them in approximately equal portions. Drink immediately.

Pine needles drink

Pine needle drink is a perfect drink made from evergreen pine needles. Select your pine needles by picking the newest green ones from a pine tree. Wash the pine needles thoroughly. Put them in a cloth bag, and steep it in a pot of boiling water—if you don't use a cloth bag, then strain the needles before drinking. Cover and let it sit for 30 minutes.

Pine needle drink is loaded with vitamin C and other nutrients to offer the following benefits: eyesight; fatigue; heart disease; kidney ailments; sclerosis (inflammatory nerve disorder); and varicose veins.

Foods to Avoid to Protect the Immune System

Sugar

A recent U.S. Department of Agriculture (USDA) survey revealed that the average American consumes the equivalent of 160 pounds of sugar a year—that is, something like over 50-heaped teaspoons of sugar per person per day.

Avoid all white sugar, corn syrup, Aspartame and Nutrasweet©. Sugar is one of the common toxic foods that stresses the immune system; it is not a health food by any stretch of imagination because it spells toxicity in many ways:

Too much sugar may suppress your immune system and upset your body's mineral balance, making it more acidic.

Too much sugar consumption may cause blood sugar imbalance and food craving, leading to obesity.

Too much sugar may overburden your pancreas, rendering it incapable of clearing sugar from your blood efficiently. This sugar imbalance may potentially lead to diabetes.

Too much sugar intake may cause anxiety, irritability, nervous tension, and even depression due to depletion of your body's B-complex vitamins and minerals, especially for those women progressing to menopause.

Too much sugar consumption may reduce your absorption of good cholesterol (HDLs), while increasing your bad cholesterol (LDLs).

Eating too much sugar is not healthy eating at all. Look at all food and drink labels before you consume them. Any food item loaded with sugar is bad for your immune system.

Unfortunately, sugar is also *hidden* in almost all commercial processed foods and drinks that are available at supermarkets.

Corn syrup, known as glucose syrup outside the United States, comes from cornstarch, composed mainly of glucose. A series of enzymatic reactions is used to convert the cornstarch to corn syrup to sweeten soft drinks, juices, ice cream, whole wheat bread and many other mass-produced foods.

Corn syrup in its liquid form not only keeps foods moist but also prevents them from quickly spoiling. It is good for food manufacturers, but bad for you. Corn syrup is not for healthy eating.

High fructose corn syrup (HFCS) is a modified form of corn syrup that has an increased level of fructose. HFCS is no more or less harmful than other forms of sugar.

Aspartame was accidentally discovered in 1965 as a sweetener.

The dangers of aspartame poisoning have been a well-guarded secret since the 1980s. The research and history of aspartame have attested to aspartame as being a cause of illness and toxic reactions in the human body. There is conclusive evidence that aspartame is a dangerous chemical food additive, and its use during pregnancy and by children is one of the greatest modern health concerns.

Unfortunately, in 1996, aspartame was finally approved by the FDA. It took decades to get the

FDA's approval for a good reason—there was, and there is, too much objection to its much controversial safety to the public health. With the blessing from the United States, now aspartame is extensively used in most processed foods and drug items, including even some nutritional supplements.

Today, millions of people around the world consume products containing aspartame. Its wide popularity is due to its low caloric value as well as its sugar-like taste. In fact, the calories in most processed foods can be substantially reduced, if not eliminated, by using aspartame in place of sugar.

<u>Suggested sugar replacements for healthy eating for a healthy immune system</u>

If you must have sugar in spite of its deadly potentials, consider the following alternatives for a healthier immune system:

- Use apple or other sweet fruit juices for many recipes in cooking and desserts. But avoid juices made from "concentrate", which have little or no nutritional value.

- Use barley malt made from sprouted barley, or brown rice syrup in bakery.

- Use blackstrap molasses, a by-product of sugar refining process, which contains calcium, iron, and B vitamins, and which has about a quarter of the calories of refined sugar.

- Use dried fruit puree made from dried organic apricots, cranberries, dates, figs, and prunes that have not been treated with sulfur.

- Use fresh carrot juice as a refreshing sweet drink.

- Use maple syrup in cooking or as a sweetener. Maple syrup comes from sap of maple tree. Organic pure 100 percent maple syrup is a little expensive but still highly recommended.

- Use raisins as a sweetener with oatmeal and fruit salad.

- Use stewed fruits as desserts.

- Use sweet brown rice with raisins as a sweet-tasting meal or dessert.

- Use vanilla rice milk to replace milk and sugar in teas and cereals

There are indeed many ways to avoid sugar in your cooking and diet. Wherever possible, avoid sugar.

Dairy products

Today's milk is no more than a *chemical*, *biological*, and *bacterial* cocktail.

Instead of the old-fashioned fresh green grass feeding and traditional methods of breeding, modern feeding methods of cows use high-protein, soy-based feeds, and high-technology breeding to produce cows with abnormally large pituitary glands so that they can *artificially* produce much more milk. Just think about *that*!

Today, an average cow may produce 30,000 to 40,000 pounds of milk per year, as opposed to the 2,000 pounds produced by its counterpart half a century ago. Such discrepancy may be due to drugs, antibiotics, hormones, forced feeding plans, and specialized breeding. In 1990, the U.S. Food and Drug Administration approved a genetically engineered hormone injected into dairy cows to make them produce more milk. However, the Canadian government and scientists challenged the safety of that hormone to humans.

Cow's milk is no longer *pure* as it was before. Just think about *what* is in your milk.

Dairy products may play a major role in the development of allergies, asthma, insomnia, and migraine headaches. At least 50 percent of all children in the United States are allergic to cow's milk, and many remain undiagnosed. Dairy products are the leading cause of food allergy, manifested in diarrhea, constipation, and chronic fatigue, although they may not be one of the causes of autoimmune diseases.

Milk also contains powerful *growth hormones*, which may play a major role in human breast cancer. Milk is a hormonal delivery system. If you believe that breast-feeding mothers deliver substances to their infants, then you should understand that milk is a hormonal delivery system, too.

Today, milk is *homogenized*, which means the fat molecules in milk are evenly distributed within the liquid milk such that there is no visible cream separation in the milk. By *artificially* changing nature's natural mechanism, milk proteins are not broken down, and are directly absorbed into your bloodstream without your adequate digestion. Undigested proteins may account for increased rates of cancers, especially breast cancers, and heart disease. This may explain why there is such low incidence of breast cancer in rural China, where there is low consumption of dairy products.

To make matters worse, *synthetic* vitamin D is often fortified and added to homogenized milk to replace the natural vitamin D complex displaced during the process of homogenization.

Synthetic vitamin D is toxic to your liver. Do not believe that your milk "fortified" with vitamin D is a better health food. No, it is not! Some good stuff has been taken out of your milk and is replaced by something not as good. For this reason, milk may not be a health food for healthy eating for everyone.

Normal milk may be bad enough as it is. On top of that, if milk is *pasteurized* (heated to kill bacteria in milk), it is being changed into something other than milk. When milk is pasteurized, much of its enzymes are destroyed in the process, making milk protein even more difficult to digest.

To protect your immune system, stay away from dairy products as much as possible.

Soy

The soybean known today is not the *same* plant traditionally grown in China. Prior to its introduction into the United States, this 20th century version of soybean was *genetically manipulated* in Europe in the 1950s to increase its yield for industrial purposes. In fact, soybean was listed in the 1913 U.S. Department of Agriculture (USDA) handbook not as a food but as an industrial product.

Soy may not be the health food for healthy eating that the food industry claims for the following reasons:

- Soy has high concentrations of certain chemicals that combine with essential minerals to deposit insoluble salts difficult for your kidneys to eliminate.

- Soy may also adversely affect enzymes and hormones production in your body.

- Soy protein is difficult for your digestion. Soybean is a seed. Like all other seeds, soybean is rich in *enzyme inhibitors* (anti-digestive) to protect it from the environment.

Soybean did not serve as a food until about 3,000 years ago when the ancient Chinese introduced the art of *fermentation*, neutralizing enzyme inhibitors and predigesting soybean with several fungus enzymes.

The Chinese did not eat unfermented soybean as they did other legumes, such as lentils, because soybean contains large quantities of natural toxins.

Only after the Chinese mastered the principle of pre-digesting soybean with natural substances to enhance its nutritional value during the Chou Dynasty (1134 - 246 B.C.) was soybean designated as one of the five sacred grains along with barley, wheat, millet, and rice for healthy eating.

Unfortunately, advances in technology, with the use of many harmful chemicals, such as emulsifiers, flavorings, preservatives, and synthetic nutrients, have turned soybean into multiple soy products, while for many centuries the Chinese have been consuming soy and its products only as a *small* portion of their healthy-eating diet.

The bottom line: consume soy products, such as soymilk and tofu, only moderately, if you *must*. Remember, soy products are no longer good for the immune system, especially your *myasthenia gravis*.

In summary, empower your mind with knowledge and information, and manage your *myasthenia gravis* with your diet and food choices, given that there is no known cure, according to modern medicine.

The TAO

According to the TAO, *extra* food is like unnecessary luggage that will not help you along the long journey of healing:

"Reaching out for it, we fall.
Running to catch it, we stumble.
Pretending to become enlightened, we become confused.
Trying to do it right, we fail.
Looking for praise, we become disappointed.
Holding onto it, we lose.

Letting go of straining, striving, and strutting, we find the wisdom in the Creator."
(Lao Tzu, **Tao Te Ching**, Chapter 24)

So maintenance means never eating more, but always eating *less* and *right*. According to the TAO, letting go plays a pivotal role in the maintenance and sustenance of your restored health:

"Letting go is emptying the mundane,
to be filled with heavenly grace.

Blessed is he who has an empty mind.
He will be filled with knowledge and wisdom from the Creator.
Blessed is he who has no attachment to worldly things.
He will be compensated with heavenly riches.
Blessed is he who has no ego-self.
He will be rewarded with humility to connect with the Creator.
Blessed is he who has no judgment of self and others.
He will find contentment and empathy in everyone.

Letting go of everything is the Way to the Creator."
(Lao Tzu, **Tao Te Ching**, Chapter 9)

Given that diet and body chemistry hold the key to maintaining and sustaining optimum health, the TAO of self-healing is just like water:

"The Spirit is just like water flowing to all things.
Its true nature is to give life indiscriminately to all.
It flows to low places, where people reject and despise.
It flows like a river, nurturing everything and everyone on its way.
Its final stop is the ocean, which is its very origin.

Living by the Spirit, we choose a simple and humble lifestyle.
We meditate to enhance our spirituality.
We love our neighbors as ourselves.
We express compassion to all.
We speak with truth and sincerity.
We live in the present moment.
We take action only when necessary.

Without much ado or over-doing, we trust the guidance of the Spirit.
In this manner, life flows like water, fulfilling itself and also everything naturally."
(Lao Tzu, **Tao Te Ching**, Chapter 8)

According to the TAO, going on with your healing journey is like frying a small fish with no worry of making mistakes:

"Living our lives is like frying a small fish;
we neither over-season nor over-cook it.

Centering ourselves in the Creator,
we have neither fear nor worry.
It is not that they no longer exist,
but that they no longer have power over us.
So, they diminish and disappear from our lives.

Walking along the Way is like frying a small fish.
We used to suffer; now we have become wise."

(Lao Tzu, *Tao Te Ching*, Chapter 60)

"A great nation is like a great man.
When he makes a mistake,
not only does he realize it,
but also admit it.
He learns from his mistakes:
everyone is his teacher,
and his enemy is his own shadow."
(Lao Tzu, *Tao Te Ching*, Chapter 61)

The Step of Restoring and Regaining

All the ancient sages and contemporary experts unanimously agree on one thing: *doing*, which involves actions and activities, is the essence of human existence. Even happiness, which is as important as health on the journey of healing, is not just about a feeling; it is more about *doing*—doing the *right* things that will make you *feel* happy.

In the same manner, you have to *do* certain things in the healing process in order to restore and regain what you have lost as a result of your *myasthenia gravis*.

Restoring Vision Lost

Weak eye muscles

Given that *myasthenia gravis* is a neuromuscular disorder, the muscles and the nerves that control vision are often adversely affected.

The muscles that create movement and vision are normally under your conscious control. However, the *involuntary* muscles (such as the muscles of your heart and many other organs, including your eyes) are beyond your conscious control. In *myasthenia gravis*, weakness occurs because the nerves that activate your eye muscles fail to stimulate them as a result of your immune cells (which normally attack foreign invaders) targeting and attacking your body's own healthy cells—known as an autoimmune response.

Double vision

If your eyes are misaligned and concurrently look at two different targets, two non-matching images will be sent to your brain. When your brain accepts and uses two non-matching images at the same time, double vision inevitably occurs—one of the hallmarks of *myasthenia gravis*.

In an attempt to avoid double vision, your brain will eventually disregard one of the mismatching images. That is, your brain will ignore one eye (called suppression).

Due to your brain's capability to suppress one eye, your double vision can temporarily go away, or its effect becomes less pronounced. However, the problem is still there. Specifically, you may gradually lose vision of one eye—the one that your brain is ignoring; in addition, you may lose normal depth perception and stereo vision.

Ocular myasthenia gravis is a type of *myasthenia gravis* that affects only the eyes and eyelid movement. The hallmark of *ocular myasthenia gravis* is eye muscle weakness that increases during activity and improves after rest.

Common ocular *myasthenia gravis* symptoms include:

- Drooping of one or both eyelids (ptosis)

- Blurred vision due to weakness of the muscles that control eye movements

- Double vision (diplopia) due to weakness of the muscles that control eye movements.

Ocular myasthenia gravis symptoms may vary in severity in different individuals.

Eye relaxation

Eye relaxation is important to *how* the eye muscles may function optimally. Eye relaxation begins with the mind *first*, and not the eye.

The mind must be *completely relaxed* before it can relax the body—and the eye, which is only one of the organs of the body.

Relax the body to relax the eye

Practicing Qi Gong, Tai Chi, and Yoga can relax the body, the mind, and hence the eye because these exercises focus on "soft" movements of the body.

Western-style exercises, on the other hand, focus more on building physical strength and muscles rather than on relaxing the muscles for total body relaxation.

Self-massage to relax the eye

Self-massage the eye for relaxation to increase blood circulation, to create a sense of ease about seeing, and to enhance eye awareness for better vision.

Do this facial and eye massage:

- Breathe deeply and slowly.

- Rub both hands to generate warmth.

- Massage your jaw with your hands moving in small circles, from the chin outward along your jawbone up to the front of and behind your ears.

- Then, move your hands over the bridge of your nose, and then massage outward along your cheekbones until you reach your temples and your ears.

- Then, starting from the bridge of your nose, massage along your eyebrows, moving above, below, and along the brow. Use your thumbs to press against the grooves slightly below your eyebrow ridge close to the bridge of your nose.

- Gently squeeze your eyeball with your fingers.

- Finally, use long, firm, strokes to massage your forehead from the left to the right, and then from the right to the left.

Throughout your facial and eye self-massage, look for sore spots, especially in the eyebrow area. Massage them with slightly harder and stronger circular movements.

Rubbing the eye

- Apply and press the heel of your left palm and the heel of your right palm against your left eye and right eye, respectively.

- With gentle pressure, rub with a twisting movement your left eye with your left palm and your right eye with your right palm.

- Meanwhile, contract and relax your eyelid muscles.

Acupressure for eye massage and eye relaxation

Apply pressure and massage from your fingers to stimulate all the acupressure/acupuncture points around your eyes.

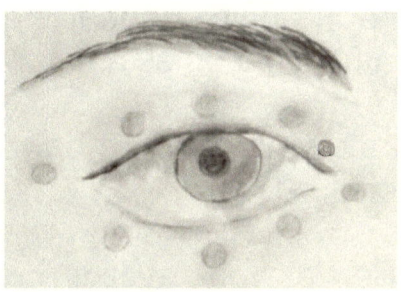

Eye exercises to relax the eye

To overcome eyestrain, which causes weak eye muscles, you need regular eye relaxation for optimum vision health:

- Consciously breathe in and breathe out through your nose to bring more oxygen to your eyes, as well as to reduce any stress on your vision. Learn diaphragm breathing and alternate-nostril breathing (see **pages 54 - 58**).

- Loosen your shoulders and keep them down to allow as much oxygen as possible to fill up your lungs as you breathe in through your nose.

- Push out as much as possible the carbon dioxide from the bottom of your lungs, feeling your stomach and chest flatten out gradually as you breathe out through your nostrils.

- It is important that you do not *force* yourself to *inhale*; instead, wait for your natural impulse to breathe in again. Repeat the process until your breathing becomes a natural rhythm.

- Concentrate your mind on only breathing and nothing else.

- Meanwhile, let your eyelids droop until they gently close. Your eyes should be *unfocused* and your eye muscles *relaxed*. Slightly open your mouth, while dropping your jaw.

- Continue breathing for a few minutes with your eyes closed.

- Now, open your eyes. When you re-open your eyes, do not focus immediately on anything in particular.

- Blink your eyes repeatedly to soothe and moisturize your eyes. If possible, induce self-yawning.

- Smile broadly and hold for five seconds to remove any tension you might be holding in your eyes.

Practice eye relaxation as often as required, especially when you feel eyestrain with *myasthenia gravis*, for better vision health.

Eye palming to relax the eye

This unique eye-relaxation exercise uses your healing hands to direct energy to your eyes, as well as to rest your optic nerve and relax your entire nervous system.

Unlike sleep, which is unconscious and passive relaxation, eye-palming is conscious and active relaxation. Therefore, eye-palming is one of the best exercises for eye relaxation. Practice palming at least for 10 to 30 minutes per session for three or more sessions daily to completely relax your eyes. Even at work, you can palm your eyes for 2 minutes, if possible, to relieve your eyestrain from the computer.

- Sit comfortably with your elbows resting on a table in front of you—preferably in a darkened room, such as a bathroom without any window.

- Rub your palms together to generate some warmth.

- Place your palms over your eyes, without touching them, while resting them on the boney ridge surrounding your eyes with the heels of your hands on your cheekbones. Your eyes should be *gently* closed.

- Relax your mind, and breathe deeply through

your nose, not your mouth. The slower your breathing is, the more relaxed your mind becomes.

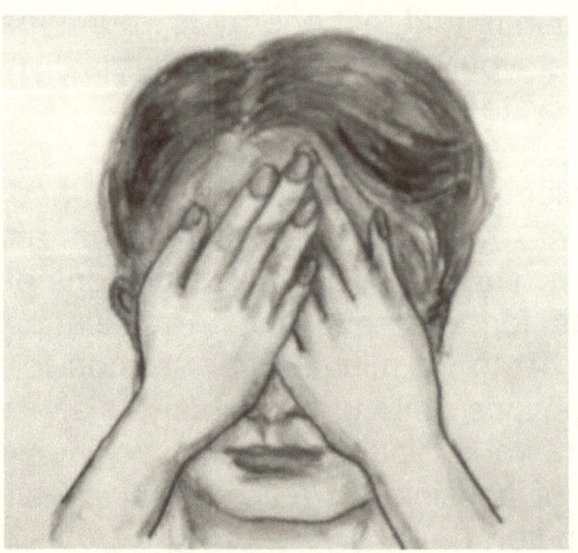

- Feel your abdomen and back expand and contract as you inhale and exhale, respectively.

- Visualize complete darkness to relax your mind.

- Feel your neck and shoulders expand and contract as your deep and slow breathing continues.

- Visualize every part of your body—hands, fingers, toes, knees, and thighs—expand and contract with your inhalation and exhalation.

Practice eye-palming whenever you feel fatigue in your eyes. It is impossible to palm for too long or for too much; some palm for hours to reap the benefits of both relaxation and meditation. If you feel any resistance to palming, it may probably be due to your subconscious mind's resistance to relaxation. If you become more relaxed, you will see *complete blackness*. However, it is all right if you do not see complete blackness; just continue with your daily palming exercise.

Remember, we are living in a stressful world, and many of us simply cannot relax, even if we very much would like to. Attesting to the inability to relax, many of us easily and often stare without blinking—and, worse, without being aware of it. As a result, our vision slowly and gradually deteriorates over the years.

The "8" eye exercise for relaxation and flexibility

Do the following "8" eye exercise as often as required to relax your eye muscles as well to increase their flexibility.

- Sit comfortably in a relaxed posture.

- Consciously breathe in and breathe out through your nose until you attain a natural rhythm.

- Imagine the figure "8" in the distance.

- Let your eyes *trace* along the imaginary figure without moving your head.

- First, trace it in one direction, and then in the opposite direction.

You can modify the exercise by imagining other alphabets and figures. The objective of this exercise, in addition to promoting relaxation and flexibility, is to train your eyes to consciously *shift* when focusing on an object in the distance, instead of eye-fixation or staring.

The Taoist squeeze-and-open eye exercise for blood circulation

This ancient Chinese exercise developed by Taoist monks thousands of years ago increases blood circulation to the eyes, prevents watery eyes, and alkalizes the eyes to detoxify the liver. It removes eyestrain and soothes eye-muscle tension.

- Inhale slowly, while squeezing your eyes tightly for 10 seconds.

- Then, slowly exhale your breath, making the sh-h-h-h-h sound, while opening your eyes wide.

- Repeat as many times and as often as required to cleanse the eyes and the liver.

Learning how to blink

If you do not blink frequently enough, you will not be able to see well. It is just that simple. Blinking has many vision benefits:

- It overcomes the harmful habit of staring.

- It relaxes the eye.

- It cleanses and massages the eye.

- It improves nearsightedness.

Learn how to blink, not *squint*. The former relaxes the eye, while the latter stresses the eye because it uses undue force to close and open the eye.

Practice the following exercise as frequently as needed to make blinking second nature to you:

- Breathe deeply.

- Close and open your eyes. The blink has to be *soft*, not hard, and it must be *complete*. Imagine using your eyelashes to cause your eyes to close and open. Practice this several times until you master it. You may even count while you blink to make sure you do not blink too fast.

- Close your right eye, and cover it with your right hand.

- Blink your left eye. If the blink is soft, and not forced, your right hand over your right eye will not feel any movement. It is important that your blinking has to be soft and effortless.

- Repeat the process with the other eye.

Always remember to blink several times before you look at something in close vision and in distant vision. Habit forming is important.

Yawning to cleanse and relax the eye

Yawning is a natural way to relax the body and the mind, as well as to cleanse the eye and the liver.

- Practice yawning *deliberately* with wide-open jaws, while expelling sounds through your mouth. If possible, induce tears from your eyes.

- After a few yawns, close your eyes, and relax.

- Now, with eyes closed, use your nose to draw the figure "8" vertically, horizontally, and diagonally (nose painting).

With practice, you can yawn *anytime* and *anywhere*, even when you are not tired.

Stretching eye muscles for relaxation

Master the eye-muscle stretching exercise to relieve

eye tension and maintain eye relaxation.

- Sit comfortably, taking a few deep breaths.

- Stretch your eyes upward as far as they can go without straining them.

- Hold your breath. Stretch your eyes downward as you exhale.

- Repeat this up and down movements of your eyes a few times.

- Stretch your eyes by moving them around in circles, but without straining them, as you breathe in and breathe out.

Perform this exercise anytime and anywhere, such as waiting for the bus, standing in line, or walking.

Softening vision for relaxation

Do the elephant-swing exercise. Practice this basic Qi Gong exercise—the elephant swing—to enhance your circulation, relaxation, peripheral vision, soft vision, and integration of vision. This is an excellent all-in-one exercise for overall vision improvement.

- Stand with your feet parallel, about 10 inches apart.

- Gently close your eyes.

- Shake your arms and legs, and roll your neck sideways, back and forth until they become soft and relaxed.

- Still your mind, and breathe naturally.

- Now, open your eyes, and look at what is in front of you. Remember not to stare.

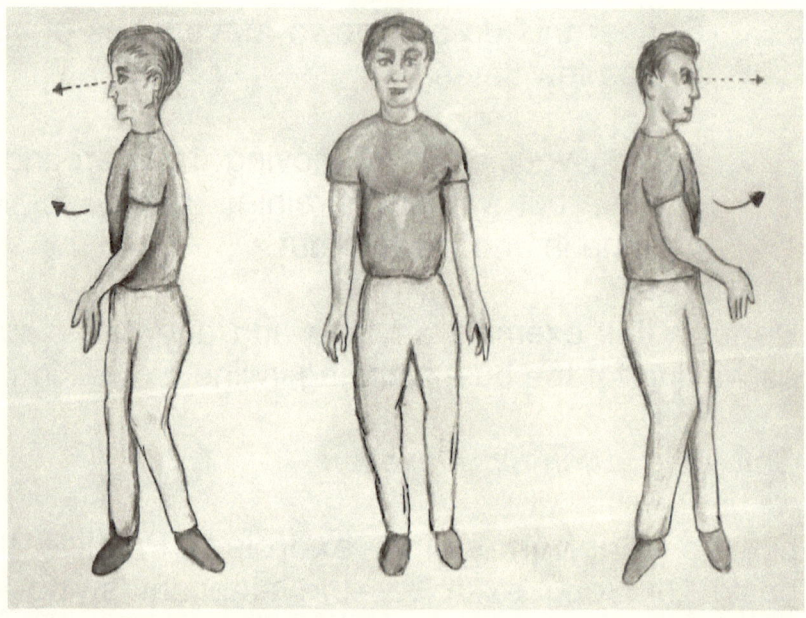

- Slowly swing your body to the left and then to the right by shifting your weight from one foot to the other and lifting the heel of each foot as you turn in a swaying motion. Let your arms hang loosely, and let your head move with your body, not by itself. The movement should be soft, natural, and relaxed, without any strain.

- Notice that the surrounding seems to "move" in the opposite direction. Let your eyes "shift" naturally without fixing on anything.

Practice this elephant-swing exercise as often as you can to soften your vision and to improve your overall vision health.

Strengthening vision

The macula in the center of the retina is responsible for detailed vision. Overuse of the central vision leads to weakening of the macula, resulting in much loss of detailed vision. This is not uncommon for those suffering from *myasthenia gravis*.

Increasing peripheral vision will decrease the use of central vision, and hence instrumental in protecting the macula and enhancing detailed vision, which is critical to good vision.

- Cut small black rectangular cards in different sizes (2"x 2"; 2"x3"; 2"x5") from construction paper. Tape the card to the top of the bridge of your nose, covering part of both eyes.

- Sit or stand, and look through the smallest black rectangular card in front of your eyes, while turning your head from side to side.

- Notice that your surrounding seems to be "moving" in the opposite direction.

- Stop turning your head, and close your eyes for a minute or two. Now, visualize the previous "moving surrounding" in your mind's eye.

- Open your eyes again, and move or wave your hands on both sides of your ears. Notice your moving hands, which are now stimulating your peripheral cells.

- Stop waving your hands, and close your eyes. Now, visualize the movement of your hands in your mind's eye.

- Repeat the above with the mid-size and then the large-size black rectangular cards.

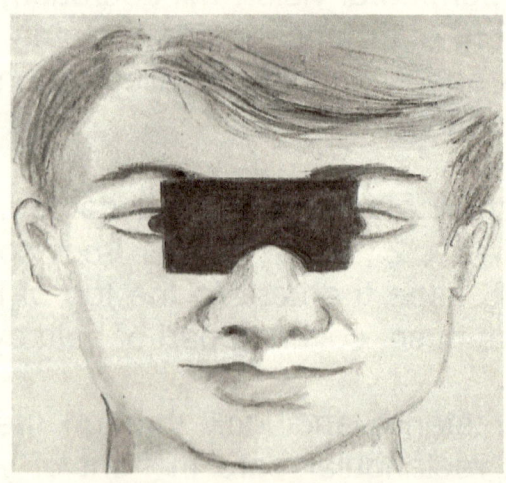

By partially covering the eyes, your mind enables your eyes to pay more attention to what is on both sides, and hence stimulates your peripheral vision.

After each exercise, you will see that your vision has "expanded" and has become "broadened." By strengthening your peripheral vision, you indirectly reduce your use of central vision, and hence protecting your macula from deterioration and degeneration.

The bottom line: regular eye exercises are critical to restoring vision and maintaining vision health, especially for those with *myasthenia gravis*. It is important to have the patience and perseverance to do these eye exercises on a daily basis. You may not see the results immediately, but the benefits are long-term.

Regaining Muscle Strength

Muscle weakness

Muscle weakness is one the major symptoms of *myasthenia gravis*. Muscle weakness, which can occur in any part of the body, may lead to progressive weakness and further deterioration due to lack of muscle use. In other words, the muscle weakness may go from bad to worse. This may result in difficulty in undertaking routine movements, setting off muscle wastage and nerve deterioration further down the road.

In *myasthenia gravis*, muscle strength returns to normal when resting. This has led many to believe that rest is the *only* option, but this is not true.

Many doctors are too willing to comply with the wishes of their patients and tell them to rest whenever they experience muscle weakness.

Research is clear on two points: oxygen deficiency (due to lack of exercise and incorrect breathing) decreases immune function; moderate amount of mild exercise increases immunity.

Oxygen plays a pivotal part in a healthy immune system. Nobel Prize winner **Otto Warburg** found the link between oxygen deficiency and the development of cancer cells. Oxygen plays a key role in your immune function because it provides ammunition for killer and natural killer T cells, as well as antioxidants.

Exercise enhances your oxygen intake and tunes up your metabolism. Both Yoga and Qi Gong conserve and generate your energy, and thus making you feel less fatigue. In addition, the rhythmic movements of these ancient Oriental exercises not only deepen your breath but also relax your muscles through the act of contracting and releasing; their postures further enhance the circulation of lymph, a fluid in your lymphatic system responsible for cleansing your immune system.

Use *soft-movement exercises*, such as Yoga or Qi Gong to overcome your muscle weakness.

Yoga

Yoga health can have therapeutic effects on muscle weakness of *myasthenia gravis* through a series of mild and easy body movements in conjunction with deep breathing techniques to enhance muscle tone as well as to reduce any physical pain. Yoga exercise practice requires neither energy nor strength. Instead, through the gentle movements, the muscles are moved, worked, and toned, with a new flow of energy into the body from the natural movements, while the enhanced blood circulation also strengthens the weakening muscles. In addition, because Yoga health is holistic health, it addresses the anxiety and fear issues of muscle weakness experienced by an individual with *myasthenia gravis*.

The bottom line: although the muscle groups may be weak, they still need to be exercised: "use it or lose it" still applies to the muscle weakness of *myasthenia gravis*. Do not let the debilitating muscle weakness overwhelm you. Instead, overcome your muscle weakness with Yoga health.

Do the following basic Yoga exercises:

- Stand with your feet shoulder-width apart. Slowly raise and stretch out both hands in front of you.

- Notice your breath, and feel the stretch along your arms and your legs (which have to be firmly rooted onto the ground), as well as around your waist. Hold the stretch for 30 seconds.

- Slowly release your arms and place them by your sides.

- Slowly rotate your head sideways, and back and forth, to stretch your neck muscles.

- Repeat the process.

The next Yoga exercise not only helps you let go of all you negative energies but also promotes your full body circulation to prepare you for the day ahead. More importantly, it can improve your body posture, which is an essential component of natural healing.

- Stand with your feet apart (shoulder-width apart), and heels turned out.

- Slowly let your body drop in front of you, with your arms loosely hanging down.

- Inhale slowly as your body relaxes further down.

- Slowly drop your chin to your chest as you release your spine, one vertebra at a time. Do not lock your knees, while slowly exhaling.

- Notice your breath, as you release your spine, shoulders, arms, fingers, neck, face, jaw, and eyes.

- Slowly return your body to a standing position.

- Repeat the process.

This third Yoga exercise not only relaxes the body, including the mind and the eye, but also massages the internal organs, such as the liver, kidneys, and intestines. This relaxed Yoga posture exercise helps you let go of all your anxieties and fears about muscle weakness, as well as stimulates the neuromuscular system to muster more muscular strength.

- Stand with your feet shoulder-width apart, and heels slightly turned out.

- Interlock your fingers of both hands behind your back.

- Inhale slowly until your lungs are full.

- Slowly lift the center of your chest, open your shoulders back, and then pull your arms down, while slowly exhaling.

- Stand firmly with the back of your knees open.

- Notice your breath and how your chest is lifted and fully open, with your arms pulled back. Maintain this posture for at least one minute.

- Now, slowly release your arms, and let them rest by your sides.

- Repeat the process.

This Yoga exercise tones your arm muscles as well as stimulates the kidneys, the liver, and the intestines to enhance internal body detoxification. By expanding your lungs, it also relieves anxiety and fear.

Given that the postures of Yoga exercise are designed to strengthen, stretch, and tone muscles and ligaments, with emphasis on particular parts of the body, you can effectively target any body part with muscle weakness. Because Yoga involves both the breath and the mind, Yoga relaxes the whole being and reduces stress, which is the enemy of *myasthenia gravis*.

Qi Gong

Qi Gong is an ancient Chinese healing art that integrates mental practice and visualization (motor imagery) into exercises for posture, body movement, breathing, and energy work. The word "qi" means "life force" or "internal vital energy of the body," and "gong" means "accomplishment" or "skill" that is cultivated through steady practice. Qi Gong is also called "the new Yoga."

The gentle, rhythmic exercises of Qi Gong mirror the movements of nature, especially the fluidity of water. In conjunction with its unique and simple breathing techniques, the ancient Qi Gong exercise is uniquely suited to strengthening not only the immune system but also the body muscles, thereby increasing the body's innate healing abilities.

Unlike some Yoga routines, the Qi Gong "flow" routines can be learned very quickly, and therefore ideal for muscle weaknesses related to *myasthenia gravis*.

Research studies have attested to the promotion of "relaxation response" by Qi Gong exercise—a phase in which your body relaxes and rebuilds, thereby instrumental in producing chemical messengers to reduce any high level of adrenal hormone to stimulate your immune system.

Therefore, to maintain some physical strength, to enhance neurological signals, and to regain some muscle strength, the mental practice of Qi Gong with motor imagery is ideal for strengthening muscles. Motor imagery, which is picturing, sensing, and feeling doing a physical action, may be instrumental in stimulating the neuromuscular system to muster more muscular strength to perform the exercise routine. According to scientific data, Qi Gong exercises can help re-wire the nervous system, creating new neurons and synapses, attesting to the benefits of the mental practice, which is a major component of the Qi Gong exercise.

Get some Qi Gong lessons from your local Qi Gong master, or watch some Qi Gong videos, showing how to move your body in a state of flow, while returning your mind to the present moment to create balance and harmony for internal healing.

Walking

Walking is also a perfect activity for those who are not well enough to pursue a more vigorous exercise. Walking is the closest to perfect exercise for those with *myasthenia gravis*, especially with muscle weakness in the legs. Studies showed that walking may have other substantial health benefits, including reducing the risk of coronary heart disease and stroke, lowering blood pressure, reducing high cholesterol and improving good cholesterol level.

Brisk is best. Brisk walking is walking without overexertion; in other words, you should be able to hold a conversation while you are walking. Of course, the intensity of walking varies according to your age and your own muscle strength. Even a 10-minute brisk walk can increase your muscle fitness, provided that it is *brisk* enough.

It should be stressed that you should also be *mindful* when you are walking. Mindfulness can add a meaningful dimension to your walking: it not only accelerates your body-mind interaction, which is critical to any healing process, but also enhances your awareness of *how* your mind may affect your body in matters of health. Do not approach walking as if you are merely performing a function of your body. Paying detailed attention to *how* you walk *is* mindful walking. Do not talk on the cell phone while you are walking.

Exercises to balance and stretch

<u>Body balance</u>

Due to your muscle weakness, especially in your legs, you may find it difficult to maintain your body balance, and therefore more prone to falling.

Find your own *focal point* by focusing your eyes on an object. Practice your body balance by slightly raising one foot, either right or left, in the following positions:

- Both hands on your hips

- Both hands at your sides

- Both hands outstretched sideways

- Both hands raised above your head in a "V" position.

Strengthen your legs for balance, equilibrium, and mobility with the following:

- Sit on a chair, and relax, with feet apart, and hands on your sides.

- Stand up a little, with legs bent, and hands on your sides, and HOLD at a count of five.

- Next, stand up a little more, with legs still slightly bent, and hands on your sides, and HOLD at a count of five.

- Now, stand up straight and tall, and HOLD at a count of five.

- Reverse and repeat the process until you sit down on the chair.

Enhance your body balance and flexibility with the following:

- Stand tall, your feet slightly apart, with your arms stretched out sideways for body balance.

- Slowly bend your right knee, and cross your right foot in front of and to the outside of your left foot, touching your right toes to the floor.

- With your right knee still bent, slowly and gently SWING your right leg from the front position to behind your left leg, touching your right toes to the floor. Use your stretched out arms to balance if necessary.

- Repeat the activity using your left foot.

Stretching

Stretching has substantial benefits for muscle

weakness: it increases your mobility range, your muscle flexibility, your energy level, your blood circulation, and your protection against injury should you happen to fall.

Wake-up stretches

Stretch your limbs before you get out of bed every morning.

Extend your arms over your head and extend your legs as far as possible until you feel the stretch in the tips of your fingers and toes. Meanwhile, inhale deeply through your nose. Then breathe out deeply and slowly while drawing your arms down along the side your body with your palms facing up. You will feel full relaxation in your legs. Repeat the stretches several times to energize as well as to relax your body.

Do a single or double knee hug. Start by bringing your knee into your chest. Massage your hip joint by moving your leg in circles in both directions. Repeat with the other knee. Finally, hug both knees into your chest, raising your nose to your knees as much as possible. Now, relax your body and let your knees fall gently down to either side. Repeat the whole process several times for stretch and relaxation.

Yoga and Qi Gong are exercises that also stretch your body and limbs to promote flexibility.

The TAO

According to the TAO, restoring vision lost and regaining muscle strength requires both "doing" and "non-doing"—*doing* what needs to be done, but not *over-doing* it, given that new beginnings are often disguised as painful endings to the many already afflicted with *myasthenia gravis*. So do not let yourself overcome by fear, worry, and anxiety in the healing process:

> "We are all desirous of making the right choices,
> fearful of making the wrong ones.
> We all pursue what others say is good,
> avoiding what they say is bad.
> We all follow the popular wisdom of judgment and preference,
> instead of the wisdom of the Creator,
> requiring us to be undesirous and unperturbed,
> just like a newborn."
> (Lao Tzu, ***Tao Te Ching***, Chapter 20)
>
> "The Way to the Creator is deep-rooted.
> Unmoved, it is the source of all movement.
> Stable, it enables us to act without rashness.
>
> So, whatever we do, we do not abandon our true nature.
> The world around us is riddled with worries and distractions.

We remain stable, steady, and steadfast."
(Lao Tzu, **Tao Te Ching**, Chapter 26)

In the healing process, you need not follow what the wise say about restoring your lost vision and regaining your muscle strength. Just be flexible and adaptable; after all, it is *your* body:

"Why then so much concern over what to say, or what to do?
Living is but an expression of the life given by the Creator.
Our true nature is a reflection of that expression.
Those who are with the Creator, the Creator is also with them.
So, success and failure are seen as part of a perfect whole.
Everything is accepted and fully lived accordingly."
(Lao Tzu, **Tao Te Ching**, Chapter 23)

Be like a baby again, with tenderness and flexibility:

"At birth, we are soft and supple.
At death, we are stiff and hard.
Young plants are tender and pliant.
Dead plants are brittle and dry.

Stiff and inflexible, we are like death.
Soft and yielding, we are like life.

Following the Way,
we become soft and supple.
That is why we always prevail,
because tenderness and flexibility
give us strength and power from the Creator."
(Lao Tzu, **Tao Te Ching**, Chapter 76)

Knowing your strength and weakness, you are well on the way to recovery:

"We do not become aggressive when we are confronted.
We do not become angry when we are provoked.
We see neither an enemy nor a competitor,
because we do not seek our own way.

Knowing both our strengths and weaknesses,
we use them to complement one another.
Thus, we find balance and harmony.
Naturally and easily, we follow the Way."
(Lao Tzu, **Tao Te Ching**, Chapter 68)

But the ultimate truths of your recovery have to be self-intuited. At the center of your being you have all the answers because you know who you really are and you then know what you really need:

"Stop striving to be righteous and wise to attain salvation,
which comes not from our efforts, not something we must earn.
Stop abiding by rules and regulations to

secure fairness and justice.
Compassion and loving-kindness come naturally to us.
Stop accumulating riches by being smart.
Heavenly assets are freely available to all.

The above are merely superficial suggestions.
The ultimate truths have to be self-intuited:
be simple, be selfless, and be non-judgmental.
Enlightenment may arrive effortlessly."
(Lao Tzu, **Tao Te Ching**, Chapter 19)

The bottom line: if you do not change your direction, you may end up where you are heading: greater vision loss and weaker muscle strength.

The Step of Balance and Harmony

After the step of regaining and restoring, the holistic healing of your *myasthenia gravis* has now begun and will continue. Given that your healing journey does not have a destination anytime soon, there will be many unexpected challenges and distracted detours ahead of you. Therefore, you need balance and harmony to enable you to continue on your healing journey.

Balance and Harmony in the Body with Balanced Foods

The Yin and the Yang diet

For centuries, the Chinese have observed the

importance of balance and harmony, manifested in the concept of the *Yin* and the *Yang* (represented as the *female* and the *male*, respectively, or any two opposing forces in Nature that balance and complement each other, resulting in perfect balance and harmony).

The terms "the *Yin*" and "the *Yang*" describe the opposite yet complementary energy states in the universe. A balance between the two polarities can help you stay in beneficial energy alignment, which is fundamental to health and wellness. The *Yin* embodies negative electrical charge and contractive energy, while the *Yang* demonstrates positive electrical charge and expansive energy.

The balance of the *Yin* and the *Yang* is reflected in the Five Elements, which form the basis of the *Yin* and the *Yang* diet for a healthy immune system.

The Five Elements

This concept of balance and harmony originates from the Five Elements (wood, fire, earth, metal, and water), which not only are fundamental to the cycles of Nature, but also correspond to the different organs of the human body. In addition, each of these Five Elements also corresponds to a different color.

These Five Elements not only balance but also complement each other to create balance and harmony. To illustrate, water nourishes trees or wood, without which there will be no fire, and without fire, there will be no earth, and without earth, there will be no metal; fire heats metal to produce water through condensation, and without metal, there will be no water. These Five Elements are inter-dependent on one another for existence in the form of a cycle of Nature.

<u>Wood corresponding to green</u>

- Eat green vegetables, from asparagus to dark leafy greens, such as spinach.

- Eat green fruits, such as lime, and melon.

- Eat pumpkin seeds.

- Eat green-colored beans, such as lentils, and mung beans; and grains, such as rye.

<u>Fire corresponding to red</u>

- Eat red vegetables, such as hot red peppers and bell peppers, or beets.

- Eat red fruits, such as red apples, or cherries.

- Eat red nuts, such as pecans.

- Eat red-colored beans, such as red lentils, and red beans; and grains, such as buckwheat.

Earth corresponding to orange and yellow

- Eat orange and yellow vegetables, such as pumpkins, squash, and yams.

- Eat orange and yellow fruits, such as mangoes, oranges, and papaya.

- Eat orange and yellow nuts, such as almonds, and cashews.

- Eat orange and yellow beans, such as chickpeas, and grains, such as corn and millet.

Metal corresponding to white

- Eat white vegetables, such as cauliflower, and daikon radish.

- Eat white fruits, such as bananas, and pears.

- Eat white nuts, such as macadamias, and pine nuts.

- Eat white-colored beans, such as white beans; and grains, such as barley and rice.

Water corresponding to black, blue, and purple

- Eat dark-colored vegetables, such as black mushroom, eggplant, and seaweed.

- Eat dark-colored fruits, such as blackberries, blueberries, and raisins.

- Eat dark-colored nuts, such as black sesame, and walnuts.

- Eat dark-colored beans, such as black beans and navy beans; and grains, such as black wild rice.

According to the famous *Yellow Emperor's Classic of Medicine*, health and self-healing are contingent on a balance and harmony of all five elemental energies. Therefore, you are recommended to eat a diet that includes vegetables, fruits, nuts, beans and grains of all the five colors in order to continue the self-healing process of the immune system to heal your *myasthenia gravis*.

The body needs balance and harmony to be connected with the mind that controls the body in the physical world.

Balance and Harmony in the Mind with Stress-Free Living

Always live in balance and harmony.

But how?

Live a stress-free life.

Stress is your body's response to increased tension.

Stress is normal. You need stress to do the following: accepting challenges; concentrating on doing a difficult task; having sex; and making important decisions.

Indeed, stress can be conducive to health. For example, sex creates stress: it increases your pulse rate and heartbeat, and stimulates your brain cells. Stress can be enjoyable, such as physical challenge in competitive sports.

But too much stress can increase your production of hormone epinephrine (and thus wearing out your hormonal glands) with the following effects: blood sugar elevation to produce more energy; breathing rate acceleration to get more oxygen; muscle tension; pulse rate and blood pressure increase; and sweating to cool down the body.

After the initial stressful stimuli, your body should be able to relax, slow down, and return to a state of equilibrium. However, if this does not happen, you become *distressed*.

Stress is the No. 1 factor not only in the cause of many human diseases, but also in the trigger of many autoimmune disease symptoms, including those of *myasthenia gravis*.

Stress and anger often go hand in hand. They cause hormone imbalance, which may trigger the development of an autoimmune disease.

Chronic stress, which causes your body to maintain physiological reactions for long periods of time, especially with respect to the release of hormones, can lead to depletion of vital nutrients in your body, particularly DHEA (a hormone critical to aging and the immune system), vitamin C, and the B-complex vitamins.

During stress, your body uses its DHEA supply and impairs the functioning of your body's hormonal glands. According to scientific research, your DHEA levels decrease with age. Therefore, stress is only adding insult to injury.

Vulnerability to stress increases with age. **Robert Sapolsky**, author of *Zebras Don't Get Ulcers*, says you lose your ability to cope with stress as you age, due to elevated blood pressure, which adversely impacts your hormone secretions, and thus creating a vicious cycle of stress and ill health.

To avoid or to decrease the symptoms of an autoimmune disease, learn to cope with your daily stress and to deal with your anger in any given situation.

The causes of stress in life

Stress may be caused by many factors, including the following:

- Money and finance

Finance is one of the main stress factors in contemporary life due to unemployment, not having enough money to make both ends meet, debt from credit cards or gambling, home foreclosure, and unexpected exorbitant medical bills, among others.

To avoid financial stress, learn how to manage your money and your daily spending.

- Health issues

    The American Academy of Family Physicians once estimated that two-thirds of all family doctor visits are stress-related.

    Health problems can be triggered by alcohol, sugar, and tobacco addiction. Chronic health problems are particularly stressful.

- Relationships

    Relationships are often a source of emotional and psychological problems, such as breakup in a love relationship, separation and divorce, dealing with teenager problems, and coping with aging parents.

- Work environment

    According to the American Institute of Stress, up to one million employees absence per day are stress-related.

Work environment creates stress due to feeling of being unproductive, inability to perform or concentrate on work, unrealistic and unreasonable demands from employers or co-workers, racial discrimination, and sexual harassment, among others.

- Special life events

    Special life events—whether they are positive or negative—can be stressful, such as marriage or a wedding, graduation, a new job, buying a home, and even going on a vacation.

Your experience of stress can be *past*, *current*, and *future*.

Past stress (also known as "residual stress") is stress from the past that you cannot overcome completely despite the passage of time.

Current stress is a current state of arousal caused by an existing situation that requires your immediate attention but that you do not enjoy addressing.

Future stress is "anticipatory stress" or worry about what "might" happen in the future. Residual stress can lead to future stress, passed on from unpleasant past experience.

The ways to handle stress

Basically, there are only three different ways to handle stress:

Relax to de-stress

Use relaxation techniques to help the body and the mind to cope with stress.

Avoid stress

Avoiding stress is only a temporary solution: it does not solve the very underlying stress problems. Avoiding stress is what is commonly known as the "fight-or-flight" response.

To deal with this type of stress, you may use your innate defensive mechanism to cope with stress by subconsciously distorting the realty. This is only tantamount to self-denial of a stressful situation.

Unfortunately, avoidance of stress only reinforces the feeling of inadequacy and therefore perpetuates the vicious cycle of stress. Avoiding or delaying the problem may only intensify the stress further down the road.

Procrastination is another form of this defensive mechanism. Unfortunately, this, too, is only a temporary measure: it does not eradicate the problem itself.

Manage stress

Manage stress by changing the perceptions of stress. Stress is always in the mind's eye, that is, the perceptions of an individual.

Stress management is essentially about the perceptions of stress. In other words, it is all in the mind's eye: what is stress to one individual may not be stress to another.

The key to managing stress is to achieve the right balance between tension and relaxation.

First and foremost, you must identify the main stressors in your life, that is, the *causes* of your stress, and *why* they stress you, and not others

Then, you adopt practical measures to cope with them.

- Change your own perceptions of stress.

    Stress is nothing more than your own perceptions of it. That is to say, it is an *attitude* or a *personal reaction* to certain events and experiences in life.

    William Shakespeare rightly said: "There is nothing either good or bad, but thinking makes it so."

    John Milton, the famous English poet, also had this to say: "The mind is its own place, and in itself can make a Heaven of Hell, a Hell of Heaven."

Given that stress is no more than your own subjective perceptions, *controlling* your own perceptions is effective stress management.

Remember, your perceptions of stress are generally based on the following: *care and value*—the more you care about something, the more stressful it is to you; *choices and options*—the more choices and options open to you, the less stressed you become; *conscientiousness*—the more conscientious you are, the more stressed you may become; *enjoyment*—the more you enjoy doing something, the less stressful it is to you; *responsibility*—the more you are responsible for the stressful situation, the more stressed you become.

- Use your subconscious energies to control your perceptions of stress or just about anything in your life.

- Learn to use positive affirmations to change any negative perception of stress.

- Use your conscious adaptive mechanism to adjust to change and to learn to see your stress in perspective. They have long-term impact on coping with stress.

Self-evaluation—Be honest with yourself: what you can do and cannot do. Never overreach yourself to create the unnecessary anxiety and resultant stress. Also, be honest with others: do not wear a mask. To foster a genuine relationship of honesty and integrity, you need to be honest with others, as well as with yourself.

Support, not withdrawal and isolation—Withdrawal and isolation may show your own inability to cope with stress. Join a social group that you feel accepted and appreciated by others; seek a confidante, someone you can confide your deepest feelings of anxiety, fear, and frustration. You must feel accepted and appreciated. Studies have shown that having a close, supportive network not only reduces stress but also promotes a healthy immune system.

The mind needs balance and harmony both to control the body and to seek guidance from the soul, which supervises the mind.

Balance and Harmony in the Soul with Alignment and Connection for Self-Healing and Self-Help

Alignment and realignment

The body, the mind, and the soul work together as a system of life energy for healing. The free flow or stagnation of this life-giving energy is dependent on the balance and harmony of the body, the mind, and the soul at each and every moment. It is this moment-to-moment alignment in the body, the mind, and the soul, as well as their alignment with one another, that creates your unique state of self-healing and self-help, which is a miracle in itself.

What is your current state of self-healing and self-help?

If you are living your life as if nothing is a miracle, most probably your body, mind, and soul are in misalignment with one another. You might feel your body is not healing, your mind is strangled with sadness and doomed to despair, and you life has little or no meaning, without a goal or purpose. On the other hand, if your current state of being is one of joy, hope, and purpose, you are living as if everything is a miracle because your body, mind, and soul are not only inter-connected, but also in perfect balance and harmony with one another.

Alignment or realignment is inter-connection of the body, the mind, and the soul to achieve balance and harmony for self-healing and self-help.

The miracle of self-healing and self-help is manifested in the spiritual wisdom of the soul that guides and inspires the mind, which controls the body living in the physical world.

Connection and reconnection

According to entropy, one of the laws of physics, anything left to itself will ultimately disintegrate, and fall apart.

According to **John Donne**, the famous English poet, "no man is an island, and every man is a piece of the continent, a part of the main."

Essentially, everything in the universe is somehow and somewhat connected, just as man is connected with one another in a subtle way. The miracle of this connection is to provide balance and harmony to guarantee their existence and co-existence, that is, their alignment with one another.

Focusing on others rather than just on yourself illuminates your soul to see its necessity to express your empathy, generosity, gratitude, and loving-kindness to others. But the challenge not to do that is as great as your innate desire to seek spirituality. Therefore, simplicity in living may enhance your spirituality and increase your strength to overcome the challenge to seek spiritual wisdom.

With spiritual wisdom, you may believe in the miracle of self-healing and self-help. You will then see that all happenings in your life are somehow "connected" for an unfathomable and unimaginable purpose, and that you can turn any bad situation into an opportunity for self-healing and self-help. Believe in the miracle that you are connected with everyone you meet in your life, and that everyone can be either your teacher or your student. In other words, there is much for you to learn from any circumstance, as well as from one another. This is the miracle of alignment and connection.

The TAO

According to the TAO, not living in balance and harmony is not living for life:

> "When there is abundance, there is lacking.
> When there is craving, there is discontentment.
> Striving for power to control and influence
> every aspect of our lives
> is the source of our suffering.
>
> Obsessed with getting and keeping,
> many of us never really live before we die.
>
> Following the Way,
> we must learn to let go."
> (Lao Tzu, *Tao Te Ching*, Chapter 75)

Letting go is adapting and adjusting any imbalance and disharmony in your everyday life and living:

> "Following the Way is like bending a bow:
> one end is pulled up;
> the other end is pulled down.
> Excess and deficiency are balanced.
>
> According to wisdom of the Way:

we reduce when there is excess;
we increase when there is deficiency.
Balance is thus created.

According to common wisdom:
we increase excess and deplete deficiency.
Imbalance is thus created."
(Lao Tzu, **Tao Te Ching**, Chapter 77)

But, given that there are too many attachments in life, letting go is not easy and it requires profound human wisdom:

"Stilling our thoughts,
our needs become few.
Following our thoughts,
our distractions become more,
and thus living in chaos.

Enlightenment is our true nature.
Meditation helps us find the origin,
and thus ending our suffering."
(Lao Tzu, **Tao Te Ching**, Chapter 52)

Attachments to the world are only distractions that lead to detours, causing imbalance and disharmony along the journey:

"The Way is easy,
yet people prefer distracting detours.
Beware when things are out of balance.
Remain centered within the Creator.

Distractions are many,
in the form of riches and luxuries.
They allure us from the Way."
(Lao Tzu, ***Tao Te Ching***, Chapter 53)

No-stress living is the way to attaining balance and harmony:

"So, we no longer argue with those who are cynical.
We stop looking for their approval.
We cease taking offense at their unbelief.
We just sow the seeds along the Way,
letting the Creator reap the harvest.

To be loved or rejected,
to gain or to lose,
to be approved or disapproved,
no longer matters to us,
when we know who we are
and who the Creator is."
(Lao Tzu, ***Tao Te Ching***, Chapter 56)

According to the TAO, living in balance and harmony is all about "spontaneity" which is the understanding of the nature of all things.

According to the TAO, spontaneity is "doing without over-doing"—which essentially means "doing without *consciously* anticipating the outcome."

In the universe, there is an all-controlling force that monitors everything. You breathe in oxygen and breathe out carbon dioxide. You eat and you eliminate. You grow, mature, and die. Spontaneity is the natural built-in mechanism in each living organism. Spontaneity creates balance and harmony, expressed in the *Yin* and the *Yang* (the female and the male). Spontaneity is the ultimate understanding of the natural cycle of all things that are beyond human control: what goes up must also come down; success is followed by failure; life forever begets death:

"The Creator creates one.
One creates two.
Two creates three.
Three creates a myriad of things.

All have their original unity
in the duality of the *Yin* and the *Yang*,
the opposite life forces that harmonize.
We experience this harmonious process
in the rising and falling of our breaths.

People naturally avoid loss and seek gain.
But with all things along the Way,
there is no need to pick and choose.
There is no gain without loss.
There is no abundance without lack.
We do not know how and when
one gives way to the other.

So, we just remain in the center of things,
trusting the Creator, instead of ourselves.
This is the essence of the Way."

(Lao Tzu, *Tao Te Ching*, Chapter 42)

With spontaneity, we become babies again, living in perfect balance and harmony with everyone and everything:

> "If we are in harmony with the Creator,
> we are like newborn babies,
> in natural harmony with all.
> Our bones are soft, and our muscles are weak,
> but our grip is strong and powerful.
> Not knowing about sex,
> we manifest sexual arousal.
> Crying all day long,
> we lose not our voice.
> With constancy and harmony,
> we accomplish all daily tasks
> without growing tired.
>
> In natural harmony with the Creator,
> we let all things come and go,
> exerting no effort, showing no desire,
> and expecting no result.
> Natural harmony is experienced
> only in the present moment,
> when we see the natural laws of the Creator."
> (Lao Tzu, *Tao Te Ching*, Chapter 55)

According to the TAO, living in the present moment is living in balance and harmony:

> "We act without over-action.
> We manage without interference.

We enjoy without attachment.

Effrontery is just
an opportunity for loving-kindness.
Great accomplishments are only
a combination of small steps.
Difficult tasks are no more than
a series of easy steps.

Therefore, we focus on the present moment,
doing what needs to be done,
without straining and stressing.

To end our suffering,
we focus on the present moment,
instead of our expected result.
So, we follow the natural laws of things."
(Lao Tzu, **Tao Te Ching**, Chapter 63)

Most importantly, spontaneity shows us the wisdom of the *impermanence* of all things—that is, nothing lasts despite all human efforts to make them continue:

"Strong winds come and go.
So do torrential rains.
Even heaven and earth cannot make them last forever."
(Lao Tzu, **Tao Te Ching**, Chapter 23)

Impermanence is one indisputable fact in life that leads to enlightenment of your *myasthenia gravis* healing. Yesterday, you had *myasthenia gravis*;

today, you are healed; tomorrow, the symptoms may come back. Therefore, the healing journey is an ongoing one; it does not have a destination.

The End

APPENDIX A

THE AUTHOR'S OWN JOURNEY OF HEALING

Many years ago, I was afflicted with *myasthenia gravis*. I was undergoing a most stressful episode in my life. I was in my late forties—call it midlife crisis if you would.

One day I felt intense pressure on both of my eyes. My first concern was glaucoma (a condition of increased fluid pressure inside the eye).

Immediately, I went to see an ophthalmologist, who subsequently referred me to a neurologist, who was. at that time the head of the neurology department in a well-known healthcare system in Cleveland, Ohio. After running some medical tests, he confirmed his diagnosis that I had *myasthenia gravis*.

My Conditions

I had developed ocular symptoms: ptosis (drooping of eyelids) and diplopia (double vision) in my *myasthenia gravis*.

In addition, my neck and limb muscles were weak,

especially on the left side of my body. I had to use a neck-rest to prop up my head whenever I drove; I could hardly use my fingers to control the mouse when I used my computer; and I could not raise my left hand without using my right hand to help prop it up. All those symptoms happened within days of my diagnosis.

Fortunately, I had not experienced any weakness of the muscles of my pharynx, which could have caused difficulty in chewing and swallowing, as well as slurred speech, in many cases of *myasthenia gravis*.

Naturally, I was devastated at the diagnosis and the conditions of my *myasthenia gravis*, which all happened within a matter of days. Worst of all, the neurologist told me that there was no known cure, although he reassured me that he could improve my disease symptoms.

Deep down, I knew it was *stress* that triggered the onset of my *myasthenia gravis*, but it was by no means the only cause. I also knew that if I did not have it then, I would probably have it further down the road. It was just a matter of time—only at that time I was not totally aware that I had been having the problem all along. I was carrying a ticking time-bomb too ready to explode on me.

Initially, I was confused and befuddled: *Why* did I get sick? For the past several decades, my health had been good, if not excellent—or so I thought. All those years prior to my *myasthenia gravis*, I had been quite health conscious in matters of foods and drinks; I had never been hospitalized all my life, and before the onset of my *myasthenia gravis*, I seldom paid a visit to the doctor. I had been having a clean bill of health up until then.

So, what was wrong with me?

I began to do some soul-searching, and looked back into my past.

Unlike most other kids, I did not have chicken pox until I was a teenager. That was a tale-telling sign that my immune system was *different* from that of others, or at least not as good as I thought it was. There was something amiss, but I did not know exactly what it was, and I could not put a finger on it.

Then, I recalled that when I was a child, I had been constantly bed-ridden with fever and coughing—my mother always worried that I could get infections from other kids, or worse, I might not live long. I was always excessively bundled up when the weather was cold.

I remember I never liked green vegetables and fish—which I would gobble up, stuff them in my mouth, and then spit them out as soon as I got out of the house. That was how bad I was when I was a kid!

As I stepped into my teens, my health conditions suddenly and significantly improved. In fact, all my symptoms of ill health disappeared soon after I had my chicken pox at the age of thirteen or fourteen. The experience of my chicken pox, however, was excruciating, but it seemed to have changed my health conditions completely for the better.

Ever since then, I had not had any major physical ailment, except that I was still susceptible to the common cold—which I often overdosed myself with over-the-counter cold medications. I did not know that all those years I had been shuffling chemical toxins into my body!

There was another episode during my young adulthood. I was frequently involved in some artwork, which required me to make some fiberglass from old newspapers by pouring some chemical solution over them. On one occasion, I accidentally mixed some toxic chemicals, giving out some toxic fume. After inhaling it, I passed out for some minutes, and I felt sick for several days.

My regular exposure to toxic chemicals in my artwork through inhalation must have damaged my immune system. Maybe the damage done was long-term and irreparable.

Nevertheless, for several decades, I had enjoyed relatively good health—or so I thought.

In my early forties, I had shingles—which was

another red flag that there was something wrong with my immune system. However, I did not pay much attention to that episode that lasted several days, during which I experienced excruciating pain.

In my late forties, the stress in my life eventually triggered the onset of my *myasthenia gravis*, which was the outcome of my over-stressed immune system.

My Treatment

At first, I was prescribed *pyridostigmine* (*mestinon*) as the usual first-line treatment for my *myasthenia gravis*.

After several months, my conditions did not improve much. I was given another prescription, *prednisone*, a synthetic hormone commonly referred to as a "steroid" medication, for my *myasthenia gravis*. *Prednisone* acts as long-term immunosuppressant aimed at suppressing the production of antibodies. Essentially, it served to stabilize my so-called "overactive" immune system.

The adverse side effects of *prednisone* for my *myasthenia gravis* included my decreased resistance to infection, indigestion, hypertension, weight gain, swelling of the face, thinning of skin, predisposition to osteoporosis, and potential development of cataracts and glaucoma.

The long list was not only depressing but also

frightening. I was worried that I would have to take all my medications for the rest of my life not just for my *myasthenia gravis* but also for the many side effects of those medications for *myasthenia graves*, such as bone loss, weight gain, and high blood pressure, among others.

In the beginning, there was some improvement in the symptoms, but overall most of the symptoms were still there, and I was never lucky enough to experience some remission from the disease symptoms.

After almost two years on *prednisone*, my neurologist, seeing that there was little improvement in my *myasthenia gravis* prognosis, switched me to *azathioprine*, supposedly with fewer side effects. That medication did not seem to have any significant effect on my disease symptoms.

My Rude Awakening

I was in a dilemma: on the one hand, I needed improvement in my neuromuscular transmission to increase my muscle strength and eliminate my double vision; on the other hand, I knew that if *myasthenia gravis* did not kill me, the many side effects of the medications eventually would.

Then, I made a decision to change drastically my diet in an attempt to discontinue my medications ultimately. The initial results of my decision were quite encouraging: I began to experience some improvement in my symptoms. Instead of gaining weight, I lost a few pounds; instead of jacking up my blood pressure, I made it plummet. I had won my first battle against the initial adverse side effects of my medications of *myasthenia gravis*.

I knew that I had to do more—much more than that. I was in for my rude awakening: there was no miracle cure for my *myasthenia gravis*; only my holistic wellness would bring about recovery and natural healing.

The Road to Self-Healing

For me, the road to recovery had been a long and winding one.

I recognized that my immune system is not only an integrated network of cells that would protect me in times of an infection, but also a system with its many regulatory mechanisms that, if uncontrolled, would become my enemy instead of my friend.

I also realized that my immune system had to be protected by being fed the correct foods, as well as being given the optimum environment free from physical, emotional, and psychological stress, which might affect my immune system negatively.

Most important of all, I began to understand that my wholesome well-being, unlike my medications that "switched" off my immuno-response when it was overactive, might hold the key to my ultimate recovery and recuperation.

My parents might not have given me an excellent immune system. I could not have chosen my parents, but I could certainly choose *my* lifestyle, and I could control what I put into my body and even what came out of my body.

I was determined to take matters into my own hands. I had to control my own health destiny.

I cherished the strong conviction that whatever my mind could conceive and believe I could also achieve.

Meanwhile, I was also fully aware of the overpowering forces of Nature. To combat Nature was futile, but I could command Nature by *obeying* it, instead of going *against* it.

> "Like water, soft and yielding,
> yet it overcomes the hard and the rigid.
> Stiffness and stubbornness cause much suffering.
> We all intuitively know
> that flexibility and tenderness are the way to go.
> Yet our conditioned minds
> tell us to go the other way."
> (**Lao Tzu**, *Tao Te Ching*, Chapter 78)

To obey Nature involved my recognition of the natural self-healing power of my physical body—if given the *right* environment.

The right environment implied that my body had to be *clean* enough internally.

Initially, I had attempted several 24-hour fasts. Finally, I decided to take the plunge: a longer fast for more than three weeks, during which I consumed no solid food, except plain water.

It was a miracle to me.

Surprisingly, I did not feel any physical weakness, not to mention any pangs of hunger. I lost some fifteen pounds. I was not overweight prior to the fast, so people were wondering if I was sick. I told them I had to cleanse myself so that I would not be sick again. Most of them did not have a clue as to what I was saying, and responded, "If you don't want to be sick, you should eat *more*, not less! Stephen, you look too thin, and not healthy at all." How could a fish explain to a bird what water is like! The internal cleansing initiated by the longer fast set the groundwork for my subsequent lifestyle changes. I was well on the road to self-healing.

Slowly and gradually, I reduced my medications, until I stopped *all* my medications, and I even stopped seeing my doctor—that happened within three to four months.

That was almost three decades ago. Now, I am in my early seventies: my blood pressure and cholesterol numbers are all normal; I am not overweight. Above all, as of now, I am not taking ANY medication at all, as opposed to taking more than ten medications a day nearly three decades ago.

Whenever I do have a health issue, I will do my best to use foods as my medicine to ultimately replace the medication prescribed by my doctor. I know that the healing journey is ongoing, and there is no destination in sight.

APPENDIX B

ABOUT THE AUTHOR

About Stephen Lau

http://www.stephencmlau.com

About His Books

http://www.booksbystephenlau.com

www.ingramcontent.com/pod-product-compliance
Lightning Source LLC
Chambersburg PA
CBHW021814170526
45157CB00007B/2592